Between Genius and Tragedy

Between Genius and Tragedy: A Psychoanalytic Portrait of Viktor Tausk offers a compelling intellectual biography and a nuanced psychoanalytic exploration of Tausk's character and thought, tracing both his theoretical-clinical innovations and the personal struggles that shaped his life and enduring significance.

Drawing on extensive archival research and newly documented material—including family sources, photographs, and testimonies made available by a direct descendant—Francisco Balbuena Rivera opens by asking why Tausk still matters. The book revisits the historical debate surrounding his figure, examining the divergent narratives constructed by Kurt R. Eissler and Paul Roazen and critically reassessing the interpretative frameworks through which his reputation has been shaped. Rather than imposing a definitive verdict, it analyses these competing accounts and invites readers to form their own judgment.

The volume situates Tausk within his familial, cultural, and intellectual milieu before offering a substantial biographical reconstruction. From the formation of his Jewish identity within the intergenerational context of the Tausk family to his immersion in the psychoanalytic movement and search for intellectual recognition, it follows the decisive stages of his development. It provides the first systematic analysis of his participation in the scientific meetings of the Vienna Psychoanalytic Society, examining both his formal presentations and his interventions in discussion. Particular attention is devoted to Freud's refusal to analyze Tausk, Helene Deutsch's failed treatment, and the circumstances surrounding his suicide.

The final part reexamines Tausk's contributions to sexuality, psychosis, repression, and defensive processes, as well as to the psychology of the deserter, situating his theoretical-clinical production within broader contemporary psychoanalytic, ethical, and philosophical contexts.

By shedding new light not only on Tausk himself but also on questions of exclusion, memory, and the politics of psychoanalytic history, this book repositions him within the Freudian tradition and will be indispensable for scholars and students of psychoanalysis, psychology, psychiatry, and twentieth-century intellectual history, as well as for psychoanalysts and culturally informed readers engaged in its ongoing development.

Francisco Balbuena Rivera, PhD, is a Spanish psychologist and philosopher and a full-time faculty member in the Department of Clinical and Experimental Psychology at the University of Huelva, Spain. His work explores the history of psychoanalysis and psychiatry, emphasizing pioneering approaches to psychosis and mental illness and their ethical and philosophical implications.

History of Psychoanalysis

Series Editor
Peter L. Rudnytsky

This series seeks to present outstanding new books that illuminate any aspect of the history of psychoanalysis from its earliest days to the present, and to reintroduce classic texts to contemporary readers.

Other titles in the series:

The Vicissitudes of Psychoanalysis in Soviet Russia, 1930-1980
Lizaveta van Munsteren

Freud's British Family
Reclaiming Lost Lives in Manchester and London
Roger Willoughby

Sigmund Freud's Inner Divisions
Personal and Theoretical
Ken Fuchsman

Sigmund Freud on the Way to Paris, 1873-1885
Foundations of Psychoanalysis
Giosuè Ghisalberti

Reading Freud's Beyond the Pleasure Principle
Trauma and Life
Herman Westerink

Between Genius and Tragedy
A Psychoanalytic Portrait of Viktor Tausk
Francisco Balbuena Rivera

For further information about this series please visit https://www.routledge.com/The-History-of-Psychoanalysis-Series/book-series/KARNHIPSY

Between Genius and Tragedy

A Psychoanalytic Portrait of Viktor Tausk

Francisco Balbuena Rivera

Routledge
Taylor & Francis Group
LONDON AND NEW YORK

Designed cover image: Viktor Tausk, Vienna, January 1905 (aged 26).

First published 2026
by Routledge
4 Park Square, Milton Park, Abingdon, Oxon OX14 4RN

and by Routledge
605 Third Avenue, New York, NY 10158

Routledge is an imprint of the Taylor & Francis Group, an informa business

British Library Cataloguing-in-Publication Data
A catalogue record for this book is available from the British Library

Library of Congress Cataloging-in-Publication Data
A catalog record has been requested for this book

ISBN: 978-1-041-20413-8 (hbk)
ISBN: 978-1-041-20412-1 (pbk)
ISBN: 978-1-003-71642-6 (ebk)

DOI: 10.4324/9781003716426

Typeset in Times New Roman
by Taylor & Francis Books

To my wife, Rosa—whose unwavering love, steadfast support, and cherished companionship have been my constant guide throughout the writing of this book.

Contents

Preface

Reading a book—or writing one—is always a journey. As readers, we are like spectators in a theater or cinema, observing from without. As writers, we become actors on the stage, inhabiting each moment from within. Having recently turned 60—what I half-jokingly call "the sixth floor" of life—I now take on this journey as an author, sharing the reflections that have taken shape in these pages.

Writing this book has been neither simple nor easy, yet the intellectual odyssey it represents has been profoundly rewarding. Beyond the intellectual challenges it has posed, the process has carried deep personal meaning, shaped by all those who, in one way or another, have contributed to bringing this work to completion. In preparing this volume, I have drawn upon archival materials that I began gathering nearly three decades ago—most notably, my personal correspondence with Paul Roazen; Ernst Federn, son of Paul Federn; and Emilio and Guido, sons of Edoardo Weiss. These exchanges, carefully preserved over the years, have opened a rare and intimate window onto the world that surrounded Viktor Tausk. They have allowed me to approach his life and legacy not only with historical rigor, but also with a sense of personal engagement—one shaped by voices that, across time, continue to resonate within the history of psychoanalysis itself.

In the course of this work, I was fortunate to correspond with Paul Roazen's surviving sons, Daniel Heller-Roazen and Jules Roazen. Their generosity brought a deeply personal dimension to this project, as they graciously shared a photograph of their father, now included in these pages. Equally enriching was my exchange with Robert Jan Maarten Tausk—known more familiarly as Rob—the grandson of Viktor Tausk. Beyond providing valuable biographical details and indispensable insights into his family lineage, he also shared photographs that have helped shape the visual and historical texture of this book. I am also indebted to Katie Lally, whose recent doctoral dissertation on Viktor Tausk—completed for her PhD in literature and read with great care in the course of my own research—significantly deepened my understanding of his life and work. Her meticulous scholarship brought to light facets of his story that were scarcely known, and others virtually unknown, particularly his literary writings and the complex ways in which Jewish identity was experienced both within the Tausk family and by Viktor himself.

It is against this backdrop of research, memory, and rediscovery that Tausk's story unfolds. Every human life—from the most seemingly ordinary to the most complex—is a singular adventure. That of Viktor Tausk was no exception. His journey, marked by intellectual brilliance, deep emotional struggle, and uncompromising honesty, sheds light on the early psychoanalytic movement—its ideals, its tensions, and its failures. This book is not simply a biography; it is an attempt to explore the existential significance of a life shaped by psychoanalysis at its origin point. I trust that readers interested in the vibrant cultural and intellectual ferment of *fin-de-siècle* Vienna—poised at the turn of the twentieth century—and in the formative years of the psychoanalytic movement will find themselves drawn into the dramatic and often tragic arc of Tausk's story.

In our current era—defined by rapid technological change, social unrest, and ongoing global conflict—some may be tempted to look back, seeking understanding in a different time. Perhaps in these pages, readers will encounter not just a forgotten figure, but a mind still capable of provoking reflection: a man whose questions remain vital—about freedom and dependence, creativity and vulnerability, and the ethical responsibilities of psychoanalytic authority.

A note on translations: Throughout this book—both in-text and in the "References"—English translations appear in brackets only when they help the reader's understanding or when the original title might be unfamiliar to an English-speaking audience. In some instances, such as the compiled writings of Viktor Tausk or the works of Sigmund Freud, I have preferred to cite the English title within the text, while listing its Spanish counterpart in the "References." Most translations into English—primarily from Spanish, though occasionally from French, Italian, or German—are my own. Any slips, inaccuracies, or tonal infelicities should therefore be read as mine alone. I trust that those more fluent in these languages will look kindly on such imperfections, knowing that they were made in the spirit of fidelity to meaning rather than form. My hope is that what truly matters—the ideas themselves and the spirit of inquiry behind them—will speak clearly enough beyond the inevitable limits of translation.

Following this, a clarification on authorship may be helpful. While my full name is Francisco Balbuena Rivera, certain earlier publications were issued under the abbreviated form Francisco Balbuena, some of which are referenced in this volume. This clarification is offered solely to avoid any ambiguity and to ensure precision in matters of citation.

In closing this preface, my hope is that the journey through this book will prove worthwhile—not only in the intellectual sense, but also in a way that touches something more intimate. Beyond facts and interpretations, this work seeks to evoke a human presence, to retrieve a voice nearly lost to time, and to invite reflection on the ethical, emotional, and existential dimensions of psychoanalytic history. If, by the final page, the reader feels both moved and illuminated—if thought and feeling have deepened in some small way—then the effort will have found its meaning.

Francisco Balbuena Rivera
Seville, Spain
December 2025

Chapter 1

Why Tausk Still Matters

From Present to Past: Reopening a Historical Debate

Some historians of psychoanalysis—and those interested in the early years of the psychoanalytic movement—may find themselves asking: Why has interest in Viktor Tausk (1879–1919) resurfaced more than a century after his suicide? I will not offer a definitive answer just yet. Instead, I invite the reader to pause and reflect, and to draw their own conclusions through a careful reading of what follows.

What I can anticipate, however, is that this book arises from a long-standing scholarly concern: the relative neglect and, at times, misrepresentation of Viktor Tausk within the historiography of psychoanalysis. This study, therefore, seeks to do justice to a complex and frequently misunderstood figure.

In pursuing this task, I have chosen to use the original Central European spelling of his name—Viktor Tausk—rather than the Anglicized *Victor*. This choice is not merely a matter of historical precision but a deliberate gesture toward emphasizing his cultural and geographical context. Nevertheless, in citations or quoted sources where the spelling appears as "Victor," I have preserved the original.

Since the publication of Roazen's groundbreaking *Brother Animal: The Story of Freud and Tausk* (Roazen, 1969), Viktor Tausk has attracted intermittent scholarly attention, mainly through a scattered series of articles and interpretative essays published from the 1970s onward. Political scientist and historian of psychoanalysis Paul Roazen (1936–2005) played a pivotal role in bringing to light archival materials and personal testimonies that had long remained inaccessible or marginalized within official psychoanalytic historiography. Yet, despite this foundational contribution, much about Tausk remains to be reexamined, reframed—and, crucially, reconsidered.

Roazen's work quickly attracted considerable attention both within and beyond the English-speaking psychoanalytic community. Just four years after the original publication of *Brother Animal* (Roazen, 1969), a Spanish translation appeared through Alianza Editorial (Roazen, 1969/1973), reflecting the growing interest in Tausk's enigmatic figure among Spanish-speaking psychoanalysts.

DOI: 10.4324/9781003716426-1

In the period between the release of *Brother Animal* (Roazen, 1969) and its Spanish translation, it is also worth noting the appearance of Kurt R. Eissler's first book on the subject, provocatively titled *Talent and Genius: The Fictitious Case of Tausk contra Freud* (Eissler, 1971), which contributed to intensifying the debate surrounding Tausk's legacy. A preliminary reading of the title suggests that Freud's alleged involvement in Tausk's suicide is a fiction—an accusation that Eissler seeks to dismantle with both scholarly rigor and deep personal conviction. The ordering of "Tausk" and "Freud" is hardly accidental; it implicitly frames the story as one of aggression and victimhood, a narrative structure that Eissler clearly intends to subvert.

Kurt Robert Eissler (1908–1999), a psychoanalyst and Freud scholar, studied psychology at the University of Vienna, earning his PhD in 1934 and subsequently an MD in 1937. After completing his training at the Vienna Psychoanalytic Institute, he joined the Viennese Psychoanalytic Society. Following Hitler's annexation of Austria in 1938 (the *Anschluss*), Eissler emigrated to the United States, settling in Chicago, where he later obtained his diploma from the American Board of Psychiatry (Yorke, 1999). He emerged as a key figure in the preservation and stewardship of Freud's legacy. From 1951 to 1984, Eissler served as secretary of the Sigmund Freud Archives, a body he helped establish, and through which he tirelessly collected and curated documents by and about Freud and his circle. His work was guided by a passionate—at times zealous—desire to protect Freud's reputation from what he perceived as unfounded or hostile interpretations. This protectiveness became particularly evident in his clashes with certain biographical researchers, especially those who challenged the official accounts of the so-called "seduction theory" or called for unfettered access to Freud's correspondence (Yorke, 1999; Gavin, 2017).

Aligned with Anna Freud (1895–1982), fervent guardian of her father's legacy, Eissler shared the prevailing deference toward her authority on questions concerning the publication of Freud's letters—most of which she firmly opposed releasing. His concern was not simply personal loyalty, but a broader fear that such material could be misinterpreted and weaponized against Freud. He insisted that only qualified and responsible editors should be permitted access to sensitive materials, with an eye toward protecting patient confidentiality and psychoanalytic ethics. Nevertheless, Eissler's restrictive approach provoked controversy. In October 1984, he resigned from the Archives amid growing disputes over access and transparency. The ensuing shift in leadership—under Professor Joseph Goldstein (1923–2000) and later Harold P. Blum (1929–2024)—moved the institution toward greater openness, leading to the eventual public release of Freud's letters (Gavin, 2017).

Eissler's *Talent and Genius* (Eissler, 1971) must be read within this broader context: a defensive gesture, born not only of intellectual commitment but also of institutional loyalties and ethical concerns. His response to Roazen was not merely scholarly disagreement—it reflected a deeper struggle over who owns Freud's legacy, and how that legacy should be narrated.

If Eissler were alive today, I would offer a suggestion: to rename his book *Talent and Genius* (Eissler, 1971) with the subtitle the difficult relationship between Freud and Tausk. Such a rephrasing would shift the emphasis away from a polemic toward a more nuanced understanding of a complex and troubled bond. As clinical experience teaches us, every human interaction is shaped by mutual influence. In the case of Freud and Tausk, responsibility was shared. Though not necessarily in equal measure, neither can be viewed as solely accountable for the deterioration of their personal and professional relationship.

Thus, rather than perpetuating binary narratives that assign blame or idealize genius, we are called to adopt a more textured view—one that allows room for contradiction, vulnerability, and emotional complexity. The Freud–Tausk story is not merely a chapter in institutional history; it is also a mirror in which psychoanalysis must confront its own internal dramas: between loyalty and dissent, brilliance and breakdown, legacy and loss.

This is precisely what underlies the title of the present work, *Between Genius and Tragedy: A Psychoanalytic Portrait of Viktor Tausk*. Earlier, I did not hesitate to suggest an alternative subtitle for Eissler's *Talent and Genius*—the difficult relationship between Freud and Tausk—as a way of exposing the limitations of an account that, for all its erudition, remains insufficiently attuned to the relational and affective undercurrents shaping their bond. My own title presses this point further. It seeks to place Tausk not as a passive casualty of circumstance, nor merely as a gifted intellect undone by his own pathology, but as a complex subject suspended in that fragile interstice where creative vitality and tragic disintegration meet. The following section will examine the deeper implications of this perspective on Tausk's life.

Reframing Tausk: Why Between Genius and Tragedy

To move beyond polarized readings of Viktor Tausk, it is necessary to adopt a relational lens—one that situates his life not only in terms of intellectual achievement but within the emotionally charged field he shared with Freud and the early psychoanalytic circle. This book is thus conceived as a psychoanalytic portrait that seeks to hold in tension both the brilliance and the vulnerability that defined Tausk's trajectory.

Rather than interpreting Tausk solely through the lens of his ideas or reducing his fate to a tragic endpoint, I aim to explore how his inner life intersected with the complex, and at times destructive, relational dynamics that shaped his involvement in the movement. The title *Between Genius and Tragedy* reflects this double register: a space of brilliance, conflict, emotional entanglement, and psychic fragility.

In contrast to this framing, Eissler refused to relinquish his efforts to place full responsibility for Tausk's suicide squarely on Tausk himself. Before addressing the clinical and historical implications of that position, it is worth pausing briefly on the symbolic charge of Eissler's title—and the revision I have suggested. In *Talent and Genius: The Fictitious Case of Tausk contra Freud* (1971), Eissler evokes a polarity that aligns Freud with genius and Tausk with mere talent. As he puts it, "the genius finds or creates the habitat he needs"—and Freud did precisely that (Eissler, 1971, p. 37). By implication, Tausk failed to do so. Genius triumphs; talent falters.

This framing is grounded primarily in an intellectual distinction, where the affective and intrapsychic complexity recedes into the background. While Eissler occasionally acknowledges the rich psychoanalytic tradition that explores the links between creativity and psychopathology, and concedes certain affective nuances in Freud's comportment, his perspective ultimately remains anchored in intellectual achievement and the fundamental architecture of psychological structure. In keeping with the conventional tendency to oppose genius and talent in largely quantitative terms—indexed by the magnitude of contributions and the breadth of accomplishments—his reading leaves in shadow the densely textured emotional life that shaped, sustained, and ultimately destabilized both Freud and Tausk. Most strikingly absent is an exploration of the intersubjective field: the subtle and often wounding interplay through which each became, in part, the other's mirror and antagonist.

Yet psychoanalysis, as I understand it, is far more than a mere theory of the mind. It offers a lens through which to examine the bonds that shape human lives—how they are forged, how they fracture, and how they leave indelible traces upon the psyche that resist simple explanation. From this vantage, it is insufficient to cast Freud and Tausk in the rigid duality of genius versus talent. Rather, they emerge as two deeply intertwined, emotionally charged figures, bound together in a relationship as formative as it was fraught. I wish also to signal, in advance, that what follows will attend not solely to their intellectual accomplishments or historical footprints, but to the inner emotional worlds that shaped and shadowed their lives—their vulnerabilities, identifications, and psychic conflicts—all of which are inseparable from the narrative of their entangled existences.

Having thus established this interpretive horizon, I turn to the heart of Eissler's argument in *Talent and Genius* (Eissler, 1971), alongside alternative perspectives that both complicate and, at times, challenge his portrayal of the Freud–Tausk relationship.

A Fractured Legacy: Eissler, Roazen, and Competing Narratives of Tausk

Having laid out the interpretive groundwork and questioned the dichotomous framing proposed by Eissler, I now arrive at the crossroads where divergent narratives about Tausk sharply collide. Nowhere is this fracture more evident than in Eissler's vehement response to Paul Roazen's *Brother Animal* (Roazen, 1969)—a work that had dared to break the silence surrounding the Freud–Tausk relationship.

Bearing all this in mind, Eissler's (1971, p. 40) central claim regarding Roazen's methodology is sharply expressed in the following terms: "The combination of omission, distortion, and failure to study the sources is in this case so breathtaking that, if I were not convinced of Roazen's ineptitude, I would have to question his good faith in view of so many errors." To support this strong accusation, Eissler meticulously examines each of Roazen's statements that could serve as evidence of imprecision, contradiction, innuendo, or factual inaccuracy—whether committed advertently or inadvertently in *Brother Animal* (Roazen, 1969).

The opening chapter of Eissler's 403-page book is accordingly titled "Questionable biographical techniques." With this heading, Eissler seeks to call into question the methodological soundness of Roazen's research and his approach to collecting biographical data. At times, it is unclear whether Eissler is genuinely pursuing historical clarity or instead seeking to discredit Roazen for sidelining Tausk's complexity and portraying Freud as morally compromised in their relationship. Although Eissler adopts a historical-biographical method in reconstructing Tausk's case, his tone often shifts from analysis to polemic, creating the impression that refuting Roazen takes precedence over offering a balanced historical account. His principal claim is that "a closer scrutiny demonstrates the untenability of Roazen's unwarranted deductions, which he puts forth as facts" (Eissler, 1971, p. 20). According to Eissler, Roazen presents a tendentious account—one in which Freud is cast as the villain and Tausk as the victim. Eissler (1971, p. 3) implies that Roazen's method echoes the cynical Roman adage: "*Audacter calumniare, semper aliquid haeret*" ["Slander boldly; something always sticks"]—suggesting that Roazen's accusations, regardless of their veracity, are designed to linger in the reader's mind and tarnish Freud's reputation by sheer repetition and insinuation.

Eissler also comments on Freud's reaction to Tausk's death, asserting that it "has been wrongly interpreted by Roazen, as well as by most reviewers, who have castigated Freud severely on that score" (Eissler, 1971, p. 17). He contends that Roazen not only misunderstood essential aspects of the case but also failed to consider crucial evidence—evidence which, in Eissler's view, substantially alters the interpretation of events. "A more reliable reconstruction of Tausk's personality than Roazen succeeded in giving," Eissler insists, "throws a new light on the formidable situation that Freud was facing in a talented pupil's severe psychopathology" (Eissler, 1971, p. 18).

In his book—a substantial work whose introduction spans pages 1 to 6—Eissler (1971) explains the circumstances that led him to undertake this critique. According to him, the person best qualified to write a critical review of *Brother Animal* (Roazen, 1969) was Max Schur (1897–1969), Freud's personal physician. As Eissler notes, Schur died just as he was preparing to engage in that task. Although he did not live to complete the review, he bequeathed to posterity a significant biographical study—*Freud: Living and Dying* (Schur, 1972)—published posthumously three years after his death and devoted to Freud's final years.

Following Schur's passing, Eissler, then secretary of the Sigmund Freud Archives, was invited to assume what many considered an intellectual and moral obligation. As he recounts:

> Since the Archives are supported financially by the contributions of many psychoanalysts, however, it was suggested, after Dr. Schur's death, that I look into what is true and what is untrue in Roazen's book.
>
> I carry out with reluctance what some consider to be my duty, because I am convinced of the futility of the undertaking.
>
> (Eissler, 1971, p. 1)

This reluctance, however, did not prevent Eissler from producing a lengthy and intricately argued work. Before proceeding, it is only fair to acknowledge that Eissler was, at the very least, a rigorously trained and deeply erudite psychoanalyst—unlike two of the earliest and most prominent reviewers of *Brother Animal* (Roazen, 1969): Arthur Koestler (1905–1983), the Hungarian-born thinker and novelist, and Maxwell Geismar (1909–1979), the American writer and literary critic. Both men approached Roazen's book as perceptive outsiders, more attuned to its literary and moral dimensions than to the complexities of its psychoanalytic substance. Eissler, by contrast, wrote from within the Freudian psychoanalytic tradition, with an insider's sensitivity to its language and internal controversies. Even so, as noted above, he readily acknowledged that Max Schur would have been better suited to undertake a critique of such scope and delicacy. In an unusual display of humility, he writes: "I never had the signal privilege of having met Freud and know little more about his life than does any reader who has studied the pertinent literature" (Eissler, 1971, p. 1). Given Eissler's official position as secretary of the Sigmund Freud Archives, this statement is striking. Despite occupying such a central role, he openly admits his limited personal knowledge of Freud's life. At the same time, Eissler conveys, in no uncertain terms, the extent of his initial reluctance to engage with the task at hand. He opens his critique with an unusually candid admission:

> If my assignment had been to comment only on what is true in Roazen's book, a short essay would have sufficed. The improbable and undocumented conclusions Roazen has drawn, the misrepresentation of information allegedly given to him, the distortion by way of omissions in quotations, the outright wrong quotations—any of these alone, and certainly all of them taken together, make this a painful book to read. It is, indeed, a book that one wishes one had not ever had to read.
>
> (Eissler, 1971, p. 2)

Despite this apparent aversion, Eissler explains what ultimately compelled him to undertake such a comprehensive response. As he clarifies:

> The only compensation I find in the ugly and wearisome necessity of having to occupy myself with it is that I have been able to place my repellent task into a broader context, which will give me the opportunity to discuss a few problems having to do with the differences between talent and genius.
>
> (Eissler, 1971, p. 2)

Yet these reflections reveal an underlying tension within Eissler himself, as he grapples with the extent to which his critique should go. He warns of the broader implications of Roazen's claims:

> Roazen's denigration of Freud culminates in an implication that, if correct, would make Freud not only unworthy of respect, but guilty of having neglected his duty and abused his standing as physician and psychoanalyst—and this for selfish, petty, and vengeful reasons.
>
> (Eissler, 1971, p. 2)

For Eissler, therefore, what is at stake goes far beyond a simple scholarly disagreement: it concerns the defense of Freud's moral and professional integrity. He closes his introduction with a passionate affirmation of Freud's character and purpose:

> Roazen has not only lured his readers, as well as future biographers of Freud, onto the wrong track, but he has also desecrated Freud's memory. Freud was a man who, despite formidable and at times even unruly passions, learned in his early years to establish in himself such discipline and mastery that he was able to harness his unique creativity to the service of mankind, and to cause only that minimal damage and pain to others without which human existence is impossible.
>
> (Eissler, 1971, p. 6)

Paraphrasing Eissler (1971), Roazen's great rhetorical gift was his "brilliance in gaining the reader's confidence and leading him by small steps to the abyss" (p. 7). As Eissler observes, Roazen constructs a "new look" of Freud's personality. His strategy, Eissler argues, is insidious: by beginning with positive affirmations about Freud's genius, and gradually introducing negative qualifiers—often undocumented—Roazen, in Eissler's eyes, manipulates the reader into accepting a distorted portrait.

Moreover, Eissler accuses Roazen of employing innuendo and subliminal suggestion, inserting emotionally charged adjectives into otherwise factual statements. The most egregious technique, in Eissler's view, is Roazen's alleged ability to "build a case where there was none" (Eissler, 1971, p. 13). The validity of this criticism is best understood in the broader context of the scholarly debate, which this book examines through detailed historical and textual analysis.

A helpful perspective on this scholarly conflict is offered by Peter L. Rudnytsky (1987), who, in note 12 to Chapter 2 of *Freud and Oedipus*—titled "The transference neurosis"—draws on Janet Malcolm's *In the Freud Archives* (1984) to illuminate the tensions surrounding the Freud–Tausk debate. Malcolm expresses strong criticism of Roazen, stating that his book is "trivial and slight" and that its scholarship "does not hold up under any sort of close scrutiny" (Malcolm, 1984, p. 7). However, Rudnytsky also notes the one-sidedness of Malcolm's praise for Eissler:

> Malcolm is unjustifiably harsh on the work of Paul Roazen, and far too uncritical in her admiration of Kurt Eissler's intemperate rebuttal. Whatever its failings, Roazen's is an important book, and Malcolm's conclusion that Eissler administers to Roazen "one of the most severe trouncings of one scholar by another in the annals of scholarly quarrelling" is so one-sided as to call her objectivity into doubt.
>
> (Rudnytsky, 1987, p. 363)

Malcolm herself characterizes *Talent and Genius* (Eissler, 1971) as "a maze of wandering thoughts, associations, notions, and meditations"— a book that reflects Eissler's complex personality, a mix of brilliance and eccentricity. His devotion to Freud, she writes, is "a kind of lovable nuttiness" (Malcolm, 1984, pp. 7–8).

Multilingual Dissemination of Tausk's Compiled Works

Despite the controversies that had long surrounded Viktor Tausk—that were reignited in 1983 by the publication of Kurt R. Eissler's second volume, *Victor Tausk's Suicide* (Eissler, 1983)—interest in his work and legacy did not simply vanish. This unwavering stance is evident in the title of his second book, *Victor Tausk's Suicide* (Eissler, 1983), where—unlike in the first volume—there is no reference to Freud whatsoever. On the contrary, as the multilingual dissemination of his psychoanalytic writings makes clear, Tausk continued to attract international attention well after the polemics had seemingly run their course.

This wide-ranging interest, reflected in the publication of his compiled works in multiple languages, suggests that the enduring relevance of Tausk's contributions transcended the biographical disputes that had overshadowed his figure. Far from being relegated to a minor footnote in Freud's intellectual orbit, Tausk's writings found renewed resonance across diverse psychoanalytic traditions—an echo of his original ambition to participate fully in the shaping of the new science of the unconscious. The very act of translating and circulating his texts across linguistic and national boundaries speaks to a broader recognition of his theoretical originality and clinical insight.

Thus, contrary to what might have been expected, with the appearance of Eissler's second book it may have seemed that the long-standing debate over the

Freud–Tausk relationship—initiated two decades earlier by the two principal interlocutors, Kurt R. Eissler and Paul Roazen—had finally come to a close. The same, however, cannot be said—as has been rightly observed above—of the broader scholarly and editorial engagement with Tausk's writings.

Indeed, interest in Tausk's work experienced a renewed momentum at the turn of that decade. In 1990, *Brother Animal: The Story of Freud and Tausk* was reissued in a second edition by Transaction Publishers, featuring a new introduction by Paul Roazen (Roazen, 1990). Since I do not possess the original 1969 English edition, but only this 1990 reissue, my references to the first edition serve merely to situate Roazen's initial historiographical undertaking.

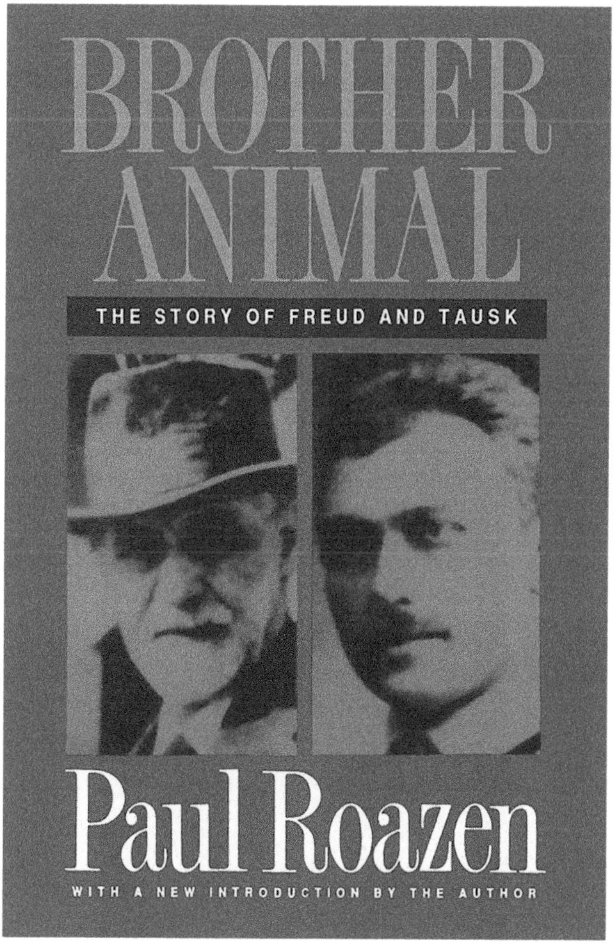

From: *Brother Animal: The Story of Freud and Tausk* (1990), by Paul Roazen. © 1990 by Routledge. Reproduced by permission of Taylor & Francis Group.

The following year, 1991, witnessed the publication of *Sexuality, War and Schizophrenia: Collected Psychoanalytic Papers* (Roazen, 1991), also edited by Roazen and released by the same publisher. The juxtaposition of these two volumes—here illustrated by their respective covers—invites reflection on how, within barely a year, the renewed editorial interest in Tausk's legacy intersected with the consolidation of Roazen's own contribution to the psychoanalytic historiography of the Freud circle.

To the best of my knowledge, this collection was reissued by Routledge in 2017 (Roazen, 2017a), retaining the English translation by Eric Mosbacher and others and including Roazen's original 1991 introduction (Roazen, 1991). Paradoxically, as Roazen himself points out in his introduction to this later edition (Roazen, 2017b, p. 5), many of these texts had long been accessible in other major European languages—specifically French, Spanish, Italian, and German—well before they appeared in English.

Within the French psychoanalytic community, Tausk's work first became available in 1975, when Payot published *Œuvres psychanalytiques* [Psychoanalytic works] (Tausk, 1975), with a preface by Thérèse Neyraut Sutterman and a postface by Jean Gillibert.

A Spanish version followed two years later, published by Granica Editor under the title *Trabajos psicoanalíticos* [Psychoanalytic works] (Tausk, 1977),

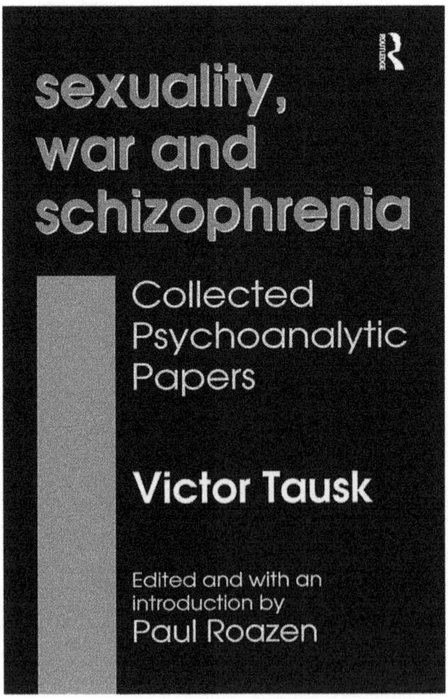

From: *Sexuality, War and Schizophrenia: Collected Psychoanalytic Papers*, edited by Paul Roazen. © 1991 by Transaction Publishers. Reproduced by permission of Taylor & Francis Group.

a title retained for the second Spanish edition (Tausk, 1983a), brought out six years later by Gedisa. It is this latter version—the 1983 Gedisa edition—that I have consulted for the present work. Accordingly, all references to *Trabajos psicoanalíticos* (Tausk, 1983a) in these pages refer specifically to that edition.

Fifteen years after Gedisa's publication of Tausk's collected writings, the only known Spanish-language monograph devoted to his figure was released. I co-authored this volume, titled *Vida y obra de Viktor Tausk: Un psicoanalista maldito* [The life and work of Viktor Tausk: A cursed psychoanalyst] (Sánchez-Barranco & Balbuena, 1998).

Our biographical volume was published by Repiso Libros, a small independent press based in Seville, Spain, which ceased operations on October 31, 2014. The edition was modest and is no longer commercially available. In contrast to both editions of Roazen's book—which feature Freud and Tausk together on the cover—our volume was designed around a singular image of Tausk, emphasizing his distinct, and often eclipsed, position within the early psychoanalytic movement.

Upon publication of this book in 1998, I sent a copy to Paul Roazen. In a warm and generous letter dated January 30, 1999, he responded: "Many thanks for sending me your fine-looking book on Tausk. It is gratifying to me that you are helping to keep the story alive!" (P. Roazen, personal communication, January 30, 1999).

An Italian edition—*Scritti psicoanalitici* [Psychoanalytic writings]—had already been published in 1979 by Astrolabio Ubaldini. The editors, like myself, opted to retain the original German spelling of Tausk's first name, Viktor, as can be verified by consulting the cover of the Italian edition (Tausk, 1979). I have chosen to follow the same editorial convention throughout this book, as I noted at the beginning of this chapter, ensuring consistency and clarity for the reader.

The German edition of Viktor Tausk's collected writings did not appear until 1983 (Tausk, 1983b). Titled *Gesammelte psychoanalytische und literarische Schriften* [Collected psychoanalytic and literary writings], this volume gathered his key psychoanalytic and literary texts. Thus, all of these translations—French, Spanish, Italian, and German—preceded the first English-language collection by several years.

Why did Tausk's key writings circulate in other European languages well before they were available in English? This remains a question deserving of careful reflection. Identifying the various editions across languages is a task that often requires detective-like persistence. Even in the editions I have consulted—the 1983 Spanish and 2017 English volumes—there is little transparency regarding how Tausk's papers were compiled and brought to publication. This editorial opacity adds a further layer of complexity for scholars attempting to reconstruct the path of his reception and dissemination.

In a gesture of intellectual honesty, Roazen addressed this issue directly in his 2017 introduction to the English collection:

> Despite the broadmindedness that English-speaking analysts like to think they have been capable of, it is only now with this book that Tausk's analytic papers have succeeded in appearing in a collected edition. If one travels on the Continent and talks to analysts today, I think it will be the case that analysts there are convinced that they are more cosmopolitan than in the United States, and the fate of Tausk's papers would support their contention.
>
> In fact, I think that most groups think of themselves as being more ideologically diverse than is in fact the case. The tale of Tausk's difficulties in remaining within psychoanalysis may have been harder to accept in North America if only because analysts here had rather more to defend than elsewhere. For although psychoanalytic ideas have been widely influential throughout the Western world, they have achieved a status and power in the United States that has remained so far unsurpassed elsewhere. Tausk's death by suicide might have been enough by itself to squelch interest in him, since psychoanalysis is supposed to be life-enhancing. In addition, there were dark rumors about his final troubles with Freud.
>
> (Roazen, 2017b, pp. 5–6)

Rather than urging anyone to adopt a specific explanatory hypothesis regarding the delayed Anglophone reception of Tausk's writings, my intention in citing this long passage is to open a reflective space. The excerpt not only highlights the complex publication history of Tausk's work, but also alludes to deeper tensions within the psychoanalytic movement—particularly the gatekeeping roles played by institutions and the enduring influence of Freud's inner circle in shaping collective memory and deciding who would be remembered and who would be forgotten.

Returning to the French context, it is worth noting that at least two articles by Jean Tréhel (2006, 2011) continued the scholarly engagement with Tausk's work in the Francophone world. This multilingual trajectory of publication and criticism underlines the uneven and layered rediscovery of Tausk—a pattern that invites further thought about how psychoanalytic legacies are constructed, transmitted, and selectively obscured.

With these considerations in mind, I invite all those inclined to do so not to passively absorb a fixed version of events, but rather to engage in a process of active and critical interpretation. This book does not seek to impose a definitive narrative; instead, it aspires to provide a forum for careful reconsideration—one that encourages us to revisit the relationship between Tausk and Freud, a bond as emotionally charged as it was intellectually generative.

In pursuit of this aim, and before asking who Viktor Tausk was—before tracing the biographical arc and existential complexities that shaped his brief yet remarkable trajectory—it is essential first to understand the circumstances in which Paul Roazen came to write and publish his influential essay. This will be the focus of the next chapter, where I examine in detail the intense resistances that erupted within the psychoanalytic establishment upon the publication of Roazen's seminal work on Tausk (Roazen, 1969). As has already been suggested in earlier passages of this opening chapter, the formidable influence wielded by Anna Freud—assisted in no small measure by Kurt R. Eissler, in his capacity as steadfast secretary of the Sigmund Freud Archives—will once again come into sharp focus.

Chapter 2

Tausk in Print

The Story Behind Roazen's Essay

Among the few scholars who undertook a sustained effort to recover and contextualize Viktor Tausk's significance—as extensively discussed in the preceding chapter—Paul Roazen stands out. For readers less familiar with his contributions, it is worth emphasizing that Roazen approached psychoanalysis not merely as a theory of the mind, but as a historically situated institution, shaped by internal tensions, mechanisms of exclusion, and shifting dynamics of power and allegiance.

Roazen's critical gaze and historical sensibility brought a necessary complexity to the ways in which we understand the psychoanalytic movement—not only as a body of theory, but as a lived and contested history. His capacity to navigate the tensions between reverence and critique set him apart in a field often marked by loyalty and partisanship.

I had the privilege, from 1996 until his passing in 2005, of engaging in a long and intellectually fertile correspondence with Paul Roazen on the subject of Tausk—an exchange that profoundly shaped the development of this study. His intellectual generosity, openness to sustained dialogue, and readiness to share archival materials, speculative hypotheses, and personal reflections revealed a mind deeply committed not only to the pursuit of knowledge but also to the ethical responsibilities of scholarship. As noted in Chapter 1, this sustained intellectual exchange ultimately culminated in the 1998 publication of a book in Spanish, devoted to the life and work of Viktor Tausk, of which I was privileged to be co-author. That collaborative achievement now stands, for me, as a testament to the rigor, curiosity, and collegial spirit that characterized our relationship. Yet this fruitful dialogue was brought to an end by his death in 2005. With his passing, the field lost a courageous and independent voice—one unafraid to interrogate psychoanalysis's internal contradictions and blind spots (Burston, 2006). Unsurprisingly, a figure of such conviction and critical acumen elicited both deep affinity and pointed resistance within the psychoanalytic community.

It is within this complex web of admiration and controversy that Roazen's scholarship—especially his work on Tausk—must be situated. The resurgence of scholarly interest in Viktor Tausk was significantly spurred by the

DOI: 10.4324/9781003716426-2

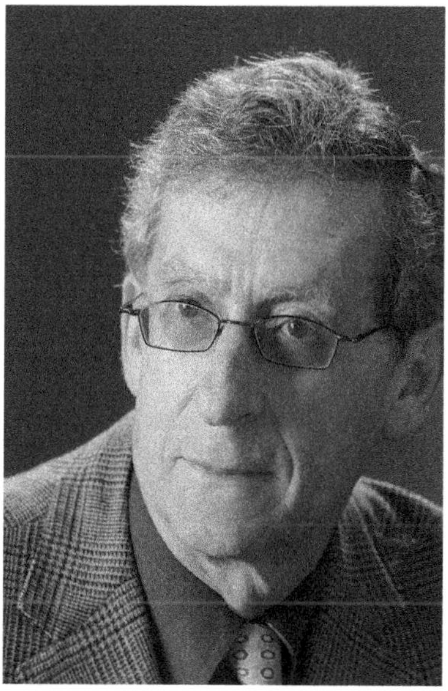

Paul Roazen, c. 1990. Courtesy of Daniel Heller-Roazen and Jules Roazen.

publication of *Brother Animal: The Story of Freud and Tausk* (Roazen, 1969), released by Alfred A. Knopf in New York. As Roazen later recounted (1972), the manuscript had initially been submitted to the Hogarth Press in the United Kingdom, but was ultimately rejected—likely due to the publisher's long-standing affiliation with the Freud family, and in particular Anna Freud, who reportedly opposed the public disclosure of certain sensitive aspects of Freud's professional relationships.

This resistance was echoed by figures such as Helene Deutsch (1884–1982)—here cited with the original German spelling "Helene," rather than the anglicized "Helen," a convention I follow consistently throughout this book—who advised Roazen to omit all references to the Freud–Tausk conflict and later expressed disagreement with key aspects of his portrayal. A stance closely aligned with that of Deutsch was articulated by Eissler, who wrote:

> Dr. Deutsch [in reference to Helene Deutsch] gave him [Roazen] all the details she could recall, when Roazen sought to find out about her experiences with Tausk before she took him into analysis and during his analysis. Helene Deutsch devoted a great many hours to conveying all she knew and thought about Freud to a person whom she judged to be a competent sociologist-historian. In so doing, she fulfilled a duty that rests on all who had the signal privilege of having met Freud, since nothing that can be known about a person as unique and eminent as he was

> should be lost to posterity. However [...] her sense of responsibility was not rewarded in kind. Regrettably, the invaluable knowledge that she had imparted to Roazen was often reproduced in such mutilated fashion and so misinterpreted that she herself was not always able to identify it.
>
> (Eissler, 1971, pp. 13–14)

Despite such objections, Roazen revisited the subject in *Freud and His Followers* (1971/1978a), originally published in the same year as Eissler's rejoinder. In this work, Roazen devoted an entire chapter to the life and fate of Viktor Tausk. That same year, as discussed in detail in Chapter 1, Kurt R. Eissler (1971) released *Talent and Genius: The Fictitious Case of Tausk contra Freud*—a sharply polemical response intended both to dismantle Roazen's thesis and to vindicate Freud's conduct. Framed as both rebuttal and restoration, Eissler's book sought to reaffirm Freud's moral authority while casting doubt on the historical credibility of Roazen's account.

As Roazen (1972) argues, Eissler made no attempt to consult Tausk's surviving relatives, who were in possession of unpublished letters and manuscripts, and instead relied exclusively on the Sigmund Freud Archives in New York, over which he held considerable institutional influence.

The intensity of this scholarly dispute reflected not only diverging interpretations of Tausk's tragic fate but also deeper tensions regarding the control of psychoanalytic memory and institutional legacy. At the heart of this conflict lay not merely a disagreement over historical facts, but a broader epistemological struggle over who held the authority to narrate Freud's intellectual and relational world.

It was within this context that Roazen (1977) asserted that Eissler's foremost concern was the preservation of Freud's reputation—a mission that, in his view, led Eissler to exercise stringent control over access to archival materials. Despite a 1951 agreement with the Library of Congress that imposed temporary restrictions on the Sigmund Freud Archives, Eissler reportedly maintained selective access well beyond those initial terms. Roazen (1978b) further argued that Eissler had granted Ernest Jones (1879–1958) privileged access to photocopied materials from the Archives during the preparation of his three-volume biography *The Life and Work of Sigmund Freud* (Jones, 1953, 1955, 1957). This act, according to Roazen, contributed to the consolidation of a historiographic orthodoxy within psychoanalytic discourse—one in which sanctioned narratives were privileged, and dissenting voices often marginalized.

These tensions surrounding archival control and historiographic authority also shaped the interpersonal dynamics between Roazen and members of the psychoanalytic establishment. Eissler's handling of the Tausk affair, in particular, was characterized by a notable lack of transparency. As Roazen (1972) observes, Eissler frequently shrouded his inquiries in secrecy—even as he publicly championed scholarly precision and historical accuracy. Efforts to gather testimony were often complicated by this atmosphere of constraint: Herman Nunberg (1884–1970), for example, initially refused to participate in any research related to Tausk, though he would later revise his stance. More encouraging was the response of Edoardo Weiss (1889–1970), Tausk's former colleague at the University of Vienna, who expressed cautious support for Roazen's project. Yet even Weiss, as Roazen recounts, was allegedly cautioned by Eissler against speaking too candidly, underscoring the delicate—and often politicized—terrain that surrounded any attempt to revisit Freud's inner circle from a critical perspective.

The reception of *Brother Animal* (Roazen, 1969) also prompted objections from other figures within the psychoanalytic community. Among them was Ernst Federn (1973), who voiced discomfort with Roazen's decision to publish in full a letter written by his father, Paul Federn (1871–1950)—a document Roazen had initially indicated would be released only in part.

My connection with Ernst Federn (1914–2007) began in 1999 through an epistolary exchange, initially undertaken with the aim of gathering both oral testimony and written material about his father, in preparation for a biography I had hoped to write—a project I was ultimately unable to complete. Yet the idea has never entirely left me; it remains quietly alive, lodged in both my thought and my heart. Over the years, what began as a scholarly correspondence slowly deepened, layer by layer, into a warm and enduring friendship—a bond that remained unbroken until his passing in 2007. A tangible sign of our mutual esteem came in 2002, when I met Ernst and his wife, Hilde (née Paar) Federn (1910–2005), in person for the first time during the IXth International Meeting of the International Association for the History of Psychoanalysis (IAHP), held in Barcelona, Spain, from July 24 to 27, under the theme *Psychoanalysis in Exile: Elements of a History*. Two years later, in 2004, I visited them in Vienna to celebrate Ernst's 90th birthday.

These personal recollections might seem, at first glance, an indulgent digression from the main narrative. Yet I include them because, at the 2002 IAHP meeting—an occasion that Paul Roazen also attended—I witnessed a quiet yet revealing exchange between him and Ernst Federn. Given my deep respect for Paul—whose generosity I have already described earlier in this chapter—and my long friendship with Ernst, what I observed left me profoundly uneasy, caught between two loyalties. That summer in Barcelona, the earlier disagreement between them had clearly not been resolved. During a break in the proceedings, I saw them standing only a few steps apart in one of the conference rooms, yet they made no acknowledgment of each other's presence. The image has remained with me, as striking for what it suggested as for what it withheld. With both men now gone, I deliberately refrain from interpreting their silence; in the absence of their own voices, to ascribe meaning to that moment would be to pass judgment *in absentia*—something I consider neither fair nor ethical.

Returning to the thread of this chapter, it is worth recalling that Ernst Federn had agreed to contribute to a scholarly examination of Viktor Tausk's work on schizophrenia—not to a polemical reappraisal of Freud's role in Tausk's death. For his part, Roazen (1978b) defended his decision to publish the letter in its entirety, arguing that historical integrity demanded it and that Paul Federn's private reflections on Tausk's suicide had been rendered with accuracy.

Yet the controversies surrounding *Brother Animal* (Roazen, 1969) did not conclude with these early reactions. In the decade that followed its publication, additional articles revisited the fraught question of Freud's potential involvement in Tausk's death, though this strand of literature would eventually fade from the center of scholarly attention. A partial resurgence occurred in the 1980s with the publication of Kurt R. Eissler's *Victor Tausk's Suicide* (1983), a volume that included noteworthy commentary by Viktor Tausk's eldest son, Marius Tausk. The release of this book was particularly unexpected, given that Eissler himself had previously advocated for ending public controversy over the matter (Eissler, 1974)—a position later revisited by Roazen (1977) in his article "Orthodoxy on Freud: The case of Tausk," published in *Contemporary Psychoanalysis.*

In his 1974 article, Eissler refrained from addressing Roazen's criticisms directly, though he thanked the journal's editor for allowing him to present his perspective. Not long afterward, however, he proposed the formation of a committee to evaluate Roazen's scholarship—contingent upon Roazen's consent—suggesting growing institutional discomfort with Roazen's revisionist narrative. In 1976, Roazen submitted a letter to the *International Review of Psycho-Analysis*, which was not published. In this letter—later cited in *Contemporary Psychoanalysis* (Roazen, 1978b)—he criticized the asymmetry in editorial treatment:

> In his inaugural editorial Dr. Sandler stated that the *International Review of Psycho-Analysis* would be "a sister journal to the *International Journal* which, when it was first published in 1920, had as one of its functions 'the defence of the pure science of psycho-analysis against various forms of direct or indirect opposition.' Psychoanalysis does not now need defending in the same way as then, nor does its 'purity' have to be guarded so vigorously."
>
> Dr. Sandler's principle seems to me a sound one. It is therefore to be regretted that although the editor of *Contemporary Psychoanalysis* offered Dr. Eissler the space for a rejoinder, the *International Review of Psycho-Analysis* did not display the same commitment to the free and open exchange of ideas by extending to me the identical courtesy.
>
> (Roazen, 1978b, p. 352)

As Neumarkt (1977) observed, the life and death of Viktor Tausk continue to provoke debate within the psychoanalytic community. While these discussions have often focused on the tragic circumstances of his suicide, they have also helped preserve the memory of a figure who longed for intellectual recognition and belonging. Some contemporaries described Tausk as altruistic, discreet, and ethically grounded; others emphasized his ambition, his contentious stance toward Freud, and his occasional tendency to appropriate the ideas of others. These divergent portrayals illuminate not only the complexity of Tausk's personality but also the deeper fault lines running through the early history of psychoanalysis—fault lines this book seeks to explore in depth.

In the next chapter, I begin to trace a more nuanced portrait of Tausk by evoking the *Zeitgeist* in which he lived, situating him within the cultural, political, and intellectual landscape that shaped his thought and, subtly yet inexorably, foreshadowed his tragic fate. Within this context, I will offer a preliminary presentation of Tausk's persona—a first glimpse of the man behind the name—outlining the vital coordinates within which his life unfolded and revealing the contours of his being-in-the-world.

Chapter 3

Introducing Viktor Tausk

Situating the Man and His Milieu

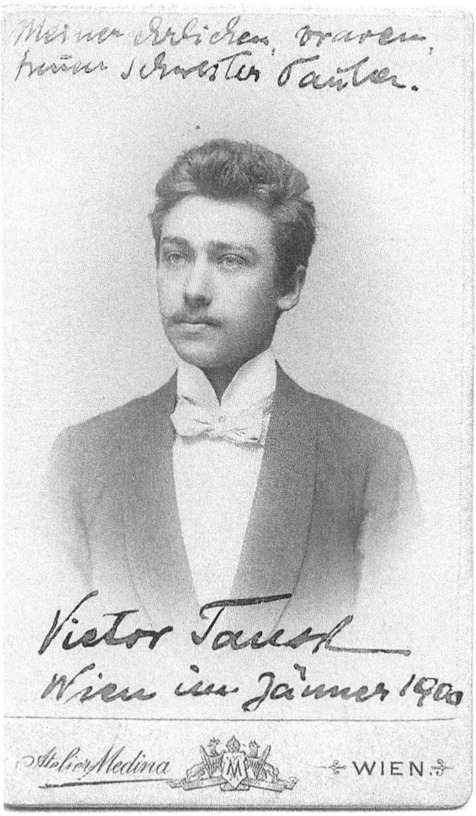

Early portrait of Viktor Tausk, aged 21, c. 1900. Courtesy of Robert Jan Maarten Tausk.

Who was Viktor Tausk? This deceptively simple question opens a window onto one of the most poignant enigmas of early psychoanalysis. Tausk remains one of the most enigmatic and intellectually compelling figures of Freud's early circle—a brilliant mind whose life and work were cut tragically

DOI: 10.4324/9781003716426-3

short, leaving us to speculate not only about what he achieved, but also about what he might have contributed had he lived longer. What theoretical directions might he have pursued? What clinical innovations might have followed from his bold insights? How might the institutional history of psychoanalysis itself have unfolded differently? The early death of Tausk—by suicide on July 3, 1919, at the age of 40—not only marked the end of a life full of promise, but also left behind a series of haunting absences. In the century since, these absences have become fertile ground for speculation, mythologizing, and selective remembrance. His legacy has been shaped as much by silence and marginalization as by his surviving texts. Understanding him, therefore, demands not only a close reading of his writings but also a careful reconstruction of the world he inhabited and the intricate interpersonal dynamics that defined it.

At a cultural level, Tausk's formative years unfolded within the broader currents of late Habsburg multiculturalism, an environment that undoubtedly exposed him to a rich diversity of linguistic, cultural, and intellectual influences. At a more intimate, familial level, however, his childhood was marked by repeated relocations, driven largely by his family's socio-economic aspirations and shifting circumstances. As I will explore in greater depth in the following chapter, these early experiences—of movement, adaptation, and negotiation between multiple worlds—must have left a profound imprint on the young Tausk. They shaped not only his evolving sense of identity but also seeded themes that would later resonate throughout his literary, philosophical, and psychoanalytic explorations (Lally, 2024).

He forged his intellectual path and emerging vocation for psychoanalysis during a time of profound transformation—a period of sweeping social, political, and cultural upheaval in Central Europe (Casals, 2003), when early psychoanalysis, propelled by Freud's creative genius and restless energy, was still defining its scope, riven by competing ambitions, and held together by alliances as fragile as they were shifting. It was within this fluid and often volatile environment that Tausk sought to make his mark. Often cast as a tragic outsider, Tausk has come to embody the unresolved tensions at the core of Freud's early circle—at once indispensable to the history of psychoanalysis and yet persistently consigned to its margins. He was a man whose personal and intellectual intensity unsettled many—perhaps even Freud himself. The circumstances surrounding his premature death, and particularly Freud's ambiguous role in the events leading up to it, continue to raise difficult questions about loyalty, authority, rivalry, and emotional complexity within the early psychoanalytic movement.

These questions, however, are not merely biographical. They speak to the very foundations of psychoanalytic theory and practice, which emerged from a highly charged interplay of personalities, passions, and politics. Within this context, Tausk's trajectory offers a privileged vantage point from which to understand both the promise and the perils of belonging to Freud's inner circle.

Originally trained in law, Tausk later transitioned to medicine—a move supported and encouraged by Freud, whose early recognition of Tausk's potential opened the doors of the Vienna Psychoanalytic Society. Once welcomed, he quickly distinguished himself as a brilliant thinker and clinician, capable of original insights and bold formulations. Yet his path within the movement soon became fraught: his emotional intensity, theoretical nonconformity, and evident hunger for acknowledgment increasingly placed him at odds with the hierarchies and sensibilities of the psychoanalytic establishment.

Tausk's relationships with key figures—most notably Sigmund Freud (1856–1939), Helene Deutsch, and Paul Federn—were marked by profound ambivalence. These were not simply professional associations, but charged emotional entanglements that shaped the course of his career and, ultimately, his fate. His drive for intellectual independence collided with Freud's mounting demands for loyalty, making him a destabilizing force within the early psychoanalytic movement—a field still struggling to establish itself as a serious alternative to conventional treatments for the mentally ill. In that struggle, psychoanalysis pushed back both against external skeptics who denied its therapeutic value and against internal voices who envisioned its theory and practice differently, seeking in both arenas the coherence and legitimacy it so urgently desired.

Within this charged atmosphere, and despite the modest size of his published work, Tausk's intellectual contributions proved strikingly original and far-reaching. He was among the first to assign psychoanalytic meaning to schizophrenic psychosis, most memorably in his seminal essay "On the origin of the 'influencing machine' in schizophrenia" (Tausk, 1919/1983a)—a text still widely cited, though too often detached from its rich historical and interpersonal context. His theoretical insights anticipated key developments in ego psychology, while his reflections extended into fields as diverse as aesthetics, law, and epistemology. Rare even within the intellectually fertile milieu of early psychoanalysis, his ability to move seamlessly between clinical observation and philosophical speculation made his work uniquely resonant and enduring.

Tausk's thought was distinguished not only by its breadth but also by its daring. He confronted without hesitation some of the most challenging questions raised by psychoanalytic theory and practice—questions of authority, subjectivity, creativity, and madness. His writings invite us to imagine what psychoanalysis might have become had it remained open to such radical, probing voices.

Building upon these insights, the following chapter turns to a more intimate terrain: Tausk's professional trajectory and the personal and familial atmosphere that surrounded him. In doing so, it lays the necessary groundwork for understanding the intellectual and emotional tensions that would ultimately shape both his work and his complex place within Freud's circle.

Chapter 4

A Biographical Sketch of Viktor Tausk (1879–1919)

Childhood, Youth, and Early Adulthood: A Troubled Identity (1879–1908)

Viktor Tausk was born on March 12, 1879, in the small Slovak town then known as Žilina. Shortly after his birth, the family relocated to Croatia, which at the time was part of the Austro-Hungarian Empire, with Vienna serving as its cultural epicenter (Casals, 2003). As Lally (2024, pp. 67–68) explains, this move was significantly influenced by the founding of the first *Matica slovenská* (1863–1875), an institution dedicated to promoting Slovak culture. Although relatively short-lived, the *Matica* fostered a flourishing of Croat–Slovak cultural relations and mutual translations, a context that likely facilitated the Tausk family's decision to settle in Croatia soon after Viktor's birth.

The growing Tausk family led a transient life across Southeast Europe—a pattern traceable not only through the publications of Hermann Tausk, Viktor's father, but also through the meticulous entries in the family's *Tanakh*, which recorded the date and place of each child's birth. According to information generously provided to me by Viktor Tausk's grandson, Robert Jan Maarten Tausk (R. J. M. Tausk, personal communication, August 31, 2025), the siblings were born as follows: Viktor (1879–1919; Jewish name: Benjamin Zeev) in Žilina, Slovakia; Ilka (Jelka) (1880–1938; also known as Ilona or Helene; Jewish name: Gittel) and Paulina (Paula) (1882–1911; Jewish name: Perel) in Ravna Gora, Croatia; Zorka (Zora) (1883–1971; Jewish name: Simcha) and Anna (Anka) (1885–1955; Jewish name: Hayele) in Koprivnica, then part of Yugoslavia; Friedrich Miroslav (Mirko) (1887–1938; Jewish name: Meir) and Vladimir (Vlatko/Vlado) (1888–1890; Jewish name: Mordehai) in Zagreb, Yugoslavia; Augusta (Guga, Gugica) (1890–1968; Jewish name: Gittel) in Ravna Gora, Croatia, as were Ilka and Paulina; and finally, Zdenko (1893–1922; Jewish name: Ichak) and Nada (1897–1983; Jewish name: Shulamit) in Sarajevo, Bosnia-Herzegovina.

Notably, neither the full list of names nor several of these biographical details are reported by Eissler (1983, pp. 6–7) and, consequently, do not entirely align with the sibling list provided by Lally (2024, p. 68). For this

DOI: 10.4324/9781003716426-4

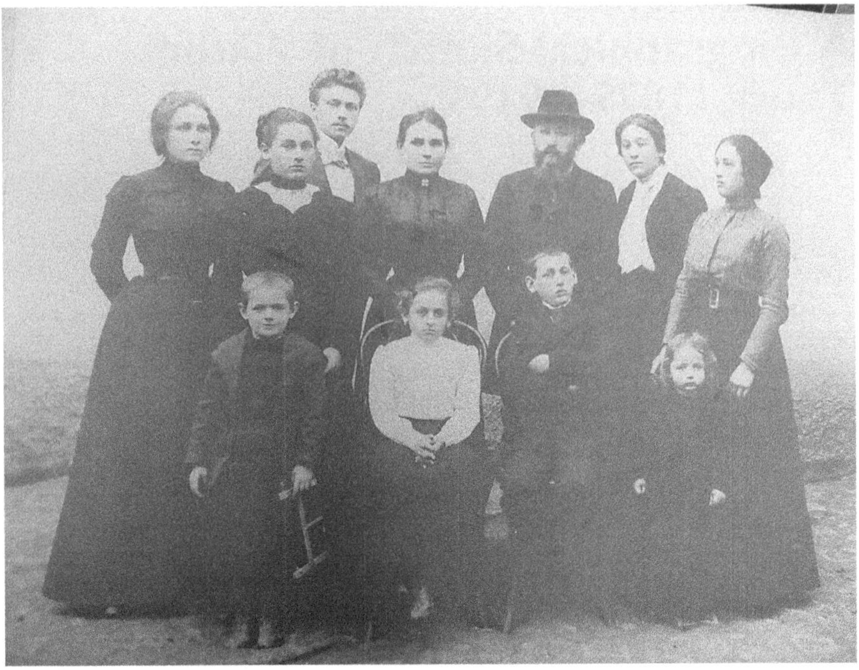

Viktor Tausk with his parents and siblings, c. 1900. Names are given as used within the family. Top row (left to right): Jelka, Anka, Viktor, Emilie "Milka" (mother), Hermann (father), Zora, Paula. Bottom row (left to right): Zdenko, Augusta, Mirko, Nada. Courtesy of Robert Jan Maarten Tausk.

reason, the most comprehensive and reliable source has been the carefully documented family tree generously shared with me, as previously noted, by Viktor Tausk's surviving grandson (R. J. M. Tausk, personal communication, August 31, 2025). Although he provided far more detailed biographical information, I will confine myself here to selected details concerning Viktor's siblings and his parents, Hermann and Emilie.

Several of Viktor Tausk's siblings endured profoundly tragic fates. Ilka (also known as Jelka) committed suicide on August 17, 1938, in response to an increasingly threatening future—a gesture clearly tied to the looming atrocities of the rising fascist regime. Paulina (more familiarly known as Paula) died of appendicitis at the age of 29, while Anna (affectionately called Anka) passed away from a femoral fracture on October 2, 1955. Friedrich Miroslav (known as Mirko), who had joined the Republican Army during the Spanish Civil War, was executed by Communist forces after criticizing their conduct (Eissler, 1983, p. 7). However, according to Viktor's grandson, Mirko's death actually occurred in 1938, when he was serving as an officer in the International Brigades and was executed alongside his girlfriend by Stalinist forces due to ideological disagreements with Communist policies (R. J. M. Tausk, personal communication, August 31, 2025). As for Vladimir (also known in the family as Vlatko/Vlado), he died at the age of 2, with no further information available. Finally, while Zdenko is noted by Eissler (1983, p. 7) to have died in 1922 of "generalized miliary tuberculosis," Viktor's grandson provides a more precise account, reporting that he died on April 29, 1922, at the Israelitisches Spital in Vienna of renal tuberculosis (R. J. M. Tausk, personal communication, August 31, 2025). These discrepancies regarding the reported cause of Zdenko's death—reflecting distinct clinical pictures and, by extension, different underlying pathologies—deserve careful consideration. This is especially relevant given that Eissler (1983, p. 6) drew his outline of Tausk's life from several sources—among them Marius Tausk (Viktor's eldest son), Wirklicher Hofrat Winter, and Franz Gall—whereas in preparing this book I relied chiefly on information provided directly by Viktor's grandson, Robert Jan Maarten Tausk. A similar divergence arises concerning the circumstances of Mirko's death, as noted earlier: depending on the source—Eissler (1983, p. 7) or Viktor's grandson—the details offered differ significantly.

Having said this, and before turning to a closer examination of the personalities of Viktor Tausk's parents, Hermann and Emilie, it is worth pausing to reconsider the question of the family's Jewish identity, which shaped not only their social position but also the broader cultural and historical context in which Tausk's early life unfolded. As Lally (2024, pp. 69–70) observes, the Tausks' relationship to Judaism was complex and multifaceted, shaped less by strict religious observance than by cultural and historical affiliations. Although their household was not traditionally religious, describing it simply as "non-practicing" would obscure important nuances. Rather than rejecting their heritage, Hermann and Emilie integrated elements of Jewish identity into domestic and personal spheres. Hermann, for instance, read and wrote Hebrew and documented the names, dates, and places of birth of each child in the family Tanakh, using both Hebrew and German. Each child also received a Hebrew name alongside their European one; Viktor's was "Ze'ev," meaning "wolf."

According to Lally (2024), Hermann seemed to conceive of Jewishness less as a religious identity than as an historically oppressed status to be politically defended. In this sense, Jewish identity in the Tausk household was deeply embedded but not strictly tied to ritual practice. This distinction between Jewishness as cultural belonging and Judaism as formal observance would profoundly shape Viktor Tausk's sense of self and intellectual orientation. From an early age, he appears to have understood his Jewish identity as interpretive rather than prescriptive—a perspective that would later influence the philosophical and psychoanalytic dimensions of his work.

It is within this broader cultural and intellectual context that we can better understand the figure of Hermann Tausk (1850–1916), an intelligent and assertive man whose professional trajectory reflected both ambition and versatility (Roazen, 1990). He began his professional career as a school-teacher but soon transitioned into journalism, a field in which he would distinguish himself through both the breadth and influence of his work. He eventually became the editor of a weekly newspaper in Zagreb, establishing his reputation as a perceptive commentator on political and cultural affairs. In 1892, likely driven by his restless and adventurous temperament, Hermann relocated his family to Sarajevo, where he assumed a central role in the Austro-Hungarian administration as head of the government's press office for Bosnia-Herzegovina. During this period, he also served for two years as editor-in-chief of the *Bosnische Post*, the official government newspaper, while simultaneously operating his own press business and working as a translator.

Beyond his official duties, Hermann Tausk cultivated a prolific career as a freelance journalist, contributing to newspapers and literary magazines across a wide geographic and linguistic spectrum, including Sarajevo, Zagreb, Budapest, Vienna, Cologne, and Bratislava (Lally, 2024, p. 87). His writings frequently reveal a deep concern for social justice and minority rights, particularly the precarious position of Jews in Europe during the late nineteenth century. While living in Zagreb, he authored a 21-page political essay entitled "Židovsko Pitanje" [The Jewish question] (H. Tausk, 1889), in which he reflected on the fragility of Jewish life and warned of the growing nationalist sentiments and emerging antisemitic tides that increasingly framed Jews as existential threats to the consolidation of new nation-states. In this essay, Hermann Tausk identified and critically dismantled the antisemitic trope portraying Jews as "mobile capital," arguing against depictions of Jews as a transnational, rootless economic force: "*da naime židovstvo predstavlja tako zvani mobilni kapital, koji ne poznaje domovine*" ["namely, that Jewry represents the so-called mobile capital, which knows no homeland"] (H. Tausk, 1889, as cited in Lally, 2024, p. 71). Throughout his essay, Hermann Tausk systematically dismantles the myth of Jewish wealth, emphasizing the economic precarity experienced by the vast majority of Jews:

> Over all, Jewish wealth is the stuff of fairytales, when for one rich Jew there are thousands of poor people, who are a living illustration of the scripture, "By the sweat of your face you will eat your daily bread."
>
> (H. Tausk, 1889, as cited in Lally, 2024, p. 71)

As Lally (2024, p. 288) observes, Hermann deliberately invokes Bereshit/Genesis 3:19, a text shared by both Jewish and Christian traditions, employing a common moral and cultural topos to reinforce his argument. In this way, Hermann Tausk anticipates theoretical concerns that Moishe Postone (1942–2018), the Canadian-born historian and social theorist, would articulate nearly a century later—particularly the antisemitic conflation of Jews with finance capital (Postone, 1980).

Taking these considerations together, and as Lally (2024, p. 71) insightfully suggests, Hermann's career was remarkably expansive, spanning multiple roles, languages, and cultural contexts:

> Hermann Tausk worked first as a teacher, then as a reporter, publisher, editor, and general correspondent for newspapers and journals whose locations of publication traced a large swath of the European continent.

His German-, Croatian-, and Bosnian-language publications appeared in outlets such as the *Sarajevski List* and *Bosnische Post* (Sarajevo), the *Agramer Tagblatt* (Zagreb), *Pester Lloyd* (Budapest), *Neue Freie Presse* (Vienna), and the *Kölnische Zeitung* (Cologne). Meanwhile, maintaining strong ties to Slovakia, he contributed as a correspondent to several Bratislava-based newspapers and literary journals, including *Slovenské noviny, Národnie noviny, Slovenské pohl'ady*, and *Obzor*. This impressive network of publications illustrates not only Hermann's intellectual reach but also his integration into the cultural and political debates of Central and Southeastern Europe during the late nineteenth century.

Yet, Hermann's public accomplishments contrasted sharply with his private persona. At home, he was known to be a strict and authoritarian father who demanded moral perfection from his children—standards he himself did not consistently uphold (Eissler, 1971). Indeed, as Roazen (1990, p. 9) documents, Hermann was unfaithful to his wife, Emilie Tausk (née Roth, 1858–1938), who was affectionately known as "Milka" (Lally, 2024, p. 66).

In a similar vein, one striking example of Hermann's double standard involved his eldest daughter, Ilka (known as Jelka), who was compelled to call off her engagement to a man she loved because Hermann disapproved. He justified his interference by claiming that the suitor had been providing child support for an alleged illegitimate child, though the paternity was never established.

Viktor's mother, Emilie, is described by Eissler (1983) as a strikingly beautiful woman with a self-sacrificing and indulgent nature. Roazen (1980, p. 2) characterized her as the archetype of the masochistic Jewish mother: endlessly generous, capable of giving up everything for others. Likely overshadowed by her husband's dominance, she nonetheless carried the burden of raising her children largely on her own, as Hermann was often absent and failed to provide adequate financial support. As a result, Emilie had to rely on her own mother for help covering basic household expenses.

According to Roazen (1990), Viktor's treatment by his parents was markedly unequal. He shared a warm and supportive bond with his mother, who took a genuine interest in his intellectual and professional pursuits. His relationship with his father, however, was fraught with tension and persistent conflict—so much so that Viktor reportedly felt uneasy being addressed by his father's surname. Lally (2024) offers a nuanced perspective on this complex dynamic, observing that, despite their strained connection, "Hermann's

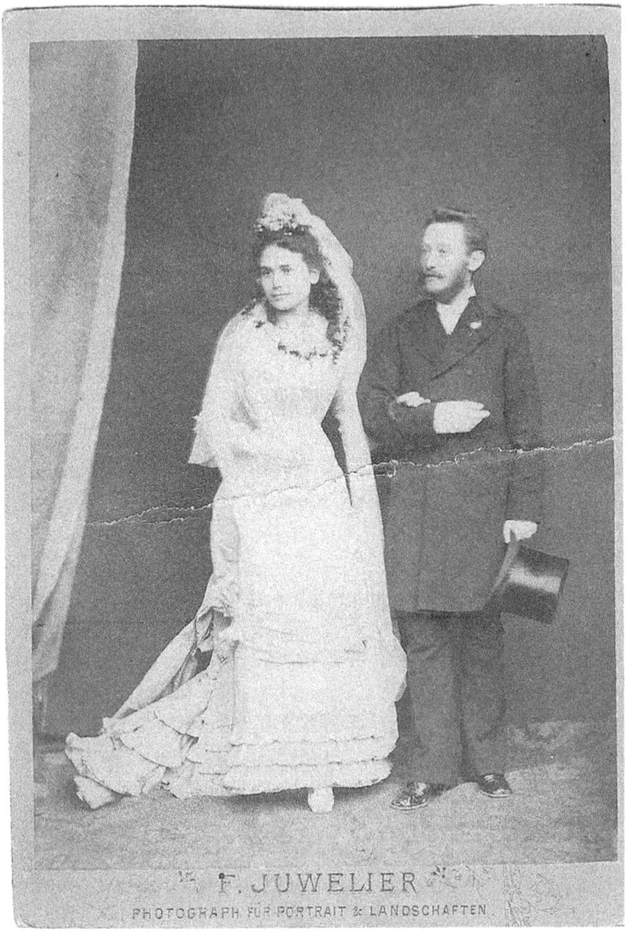

Hermann Tausk and Emilie Roth, parents of Viktor Tausk, on their wedding day, Zsilina (now Žilina), March 5, 1878. Courtesy of Robert Jan Maarten Tausk.

convictions and connections were formative to Viktor's early worldview and his literary and political milieu, whether by way of Viktor's acceptance or rejection of them" (p. 67).

Yet even with his mother, Viktor's emotions were ambivalent and conflicted. In one telling childhood episode, he symbolically "attacked" her by stabbing the heart in her portrait with a needle—an act of fantasy that, according to later accounts, left him deeply anxious and guilt-ridden. Later, when Emilie noticed that her portrait had been damaged and asked who was responsible, Viktor realized that he had not physically harmed his mother—the aggression had been directed at her image, and the murderous impulse had remained in fantasy (Andreas-Salomé, 1958/1984).

Until recently, information about Viktor Tausk's school years had remained fragmentary. However, thanks to the meticulous archival research conducted by Lally (2024, p. 83), this significant gap has now been substantially clarified. Drawing from Viktor's surviving report cards, Lally reconstructs the trajectory of his early education with remarkable precision. According to these records, Viktor began his studies at the Gymnasium in Zagreb at the start of the 1889/1890 academic year, transferring later that same year to a Gymnasium in Sarajevo. He then spent the 1890/1891 academic year at the Gymnasium in Rijeka—located on the northern Adriatic coast—before continuing his studies in Varaždin (northeastern Croatia) during 1891/1892, where he ultimately earned his *matura* degree.

Throughout this period, Viktor distinguished himself as an exceptionally gifted student, particularly in languages, mastering Latin, Greek, Croatian, German, French, and Italian. His overall academic performance was consistently strong, with the notable exception of religious instruction, where his grades were comparatively lower—a detail that resonates with the Tausk family's complex relationship to Judaism. Moreover, as Lally (2024) highlights, Viktor's school records and personal writings reveal the early emergence of two enduring traits: a rebellious independence of spirit and a profound sense of justice, qualities that would later shape both his intellectual trajectory and his psychoanalytic contributions.

It was precisely during this period that Tausk's rebellious temperament and acute sense of justice began to emerge. As Rodrigué (1996) contends, he embodied the prototype of the romantic, politicized student leader. A striking example occurred during a heated confrontation with his religion teacher: a staunch atheist, Viktor openly challenged the teacher's dogmatic views and went so far as to lead a student strike demanding freedom of thought. The ensuing conflict ultimately forced him to transfer to Varaždin, where he successfully completed his final secondary examinations. This rigorous, week-long process required students to demonstrate both oral and written mastery of multiple disciplines before their school principal and a government official. Those who passed were celebrated with a ceremonial beer toast—an event that, as Sterba (1985, p. 14) evocatively notes, echoed initiation rites observed in certain tribal societies.

After completing his Gymnasium studies in 1897, Viktor Tausk entered a period of profound transformation, marked by both personal challenges and intellectual breakthroughs. Around this time, he contracted pulmonary tuberculosis, an illness that initially threatened his health but from which he eventually made what seemed to be a promising recovery (Roazen, 1990). With renewed energy, Tausk moved to Vienna later that year, where he enrolled in the Faculty of Law. Although his true vocation was medicine, financial considerations made law the more accessible path, and he pursued it despite his lack of enthusiasm.

Concurrently, the years 1897–1898 marked the beginning of an intensely productive literary and intellectual phase that would decisively shape his later development. Even before his relocation to Vienna, Viktor Tausk had begun publishing under the pseudonym Vladoje Slovačić in Sarajevo's vibrant literary circles (Donat, 2007; Lally, 2024, p. 87). Under this name, Viktor Tausk (Slovačić) published several lyric poems in *Nada: pouci, zabavi i umjetnosti* [Hope: Learning, entertainment, and the arts], a Sarajevo-based literary journal issued twice monthly from 1895 to 1903 under the editorship of poet Silvije Strahimir Kranjčević (1865–1908), a close friend of Hermann Tausk and one of Viktor's earliest literary mentors. *Nada* was distinctive in both form and ambition: printed in both Roman and Cyrillic scripts, the journal sought to represent a heterogeneous South Slavic cultural identity through literature, visual arts, and travel writing, while also situating its contributors within broader European intellectual currents.

Among Viktor Tausk's early publications in *Nada* under the pseudonym Vladoje Slovačić were the poems "Sivo oko" [Gray eye] (Tausk, 1897) and "Zimsko cvijeće" [Winter flowers] (Tausk, 1898a), both of which employ nature imagery as extended metaphors for unrequited love while subtly gesturing toward mortality. As Petlevski (2011) comments, in "Gray eye" the lyric voice transforms an encounter with a young woman, symbolized synecdochically through "the eye," into an encounter with an elemental force of nature, blending folkloric traditions with an emergent modernist sensibility. He argues further that, at this stage, the young Viktor Tausk still believed in "the parallel, harmonious development of man and society" and viewed introspection as a pathway to illuminating "the labyrinth of social entanglements" (Petlevski, 2011, p. 71). However, Petlevski also notes that this youthful confidence would not endure. Soon, it gave way to skepticism and rebellion against authority—social, religious, familial, and literary—which, in later decades, extended into his challenges to scientific and psychoanalytic orthodoxy itself. In this sense, the trajectory from *Vladoje Slovačić* to the psychoanalyst Viktor Tausk already contained the seeds of his later intellectual restlessness.

This intersection of literature and politics also positioned Tausk within the broader emergence of Croatian modernism. As Donat (2007) demonstrates, Viktor Tausk holds a central position in linking the early modernist movements of Zagreb, Sarajevo, and Vienna with those developing elsewhere in Europe. After moving to Vienna in 1897 to study law, he remained deeply engaged with South Slavic literary networks, contributing to *Nada* and joining the student society *Zvonimir*, a hub for young Croatian modernists. By 1898, he had become one of the founding members of *Mladost: smotra za modernu književnost i umjetnost* [Youth: Review for modern literature and art], an avant-garde magazine jointly edited between Zagreb and Vienna with an explicitly international orientation (Lally, 2024, p. 104).

During this period, Tausk again published under the pseudonym Vladoje Slovačić his most radical literary statement: an 18-page pamphlet entitled "A. Tresić-Pavičić kao liričar: Studija" [Dr. Ante Tresić Pavičić as a lyricist: A study] (Tausk, 1898b), a sharp critique of the poet Tresić-Pavičić and an implicit manifesto of Croatian modernism. Ambitiously announced as the first in a planned series, the pamphlet would remain the only one published—a telling marker of Viktor Tausk's bold ambitions and the political stakes of his early literary activity. In retrospect, these early writings reveal a young intellectual already navigating questions of identity, belonging, and authority—themes that would later resurface with striking force in his psychoanalytic contributions.

At this formative stage, Tausk occupied a pivotal juncture in his personal and intellectual development: a young law student in Vienna, an emerging voice within Croatian modernism, and an active participant in the intellectual ferment of a cosmopolitan, multicultural milieu. His early literary writings, far from being a youthful diversion, already foreshadowed the theoretical concerns that would later define his psychoanalytic investigations—the dynamic interplay between the individual psyche, social identity, and the cultural-technological transformations of modernity.

It was precisely within this context of intense intellectual engagement that, in 1898, a year after settling in Vienna, Viktor Tausk's personal life took a decisive turn when he met Martha Frisch (1881–1957). Although she has long been known in the literature simply as *Martha Frisch*, family records confirm that her full name was *Martha Rosa Frisch* (R. J. M. Tausk, personal communication, August 31, 2025). For clarity and consistency, I refer to her throughout this book simply as Martha. The couple married on May 13, 1900, a date also verified by the same source. An educated and politically active socialist, Martha became formally involved with the Social Democratic Party of Austria in 1911 and, by 1918—even before women had obtained the right to vote—was elected as a member of the Styrian Provisional Provincial Assembly (Dorfer, 2007).

Martha described her upbringing as follows: "*Vater Jude, Mutter Tschechin, Erziehung in Wien, kosmopolitisch, immerhin gewachsen mit deutschem Gedankengut*" ["Jewish father, Czech mother, raised in Vienna, cosmopolitan, yet shaped by German intellectual traditions"] (Dorfer, 2007, p. 8). In her feminist-interpretive analysis of Martha Tausk's life, Dorfer situates her personal trajectory within the broader struggles for social democracy and women's rights, highlighting the formative influence of both her family and her education on her later political engagement and intellectual development. In this context, the author underscores the prominent position of Martha's father, a self-made businessman who operated a successful Viennese press, thereby exposing the family to leading authors, political thinkers, and the vibrant cultural debates of the era. Martha's intellectual formation was further enriched by her personal and familial connections to prominent figures: she maintained a close childhood friendship with the future physicist Lise Meitner (1878–1968) and was a cousin of the Jewish philosopher Martin Buber (1878–1965) through her paternal aunt, Marie Frisch (Lally, 2024, p. 103). As Rodrigué (1996) remarks, Martha embodied the archetype of the radical feminist Marxist of her time, rejecting conventional aesthetics—including shaving and deodorant—as political statements. Martha's family disapproved of the engagement, citing irreconcilable psychological differences between Viktor and her father. Nevertheless, the two married in 1900 under Protestant rites, after Martha became pregnant. To make the ceremony possible, Viktor had to be baptized—though he concealed this fact, never renouncing his Jewish identity and remaining, in practice, an atheist.

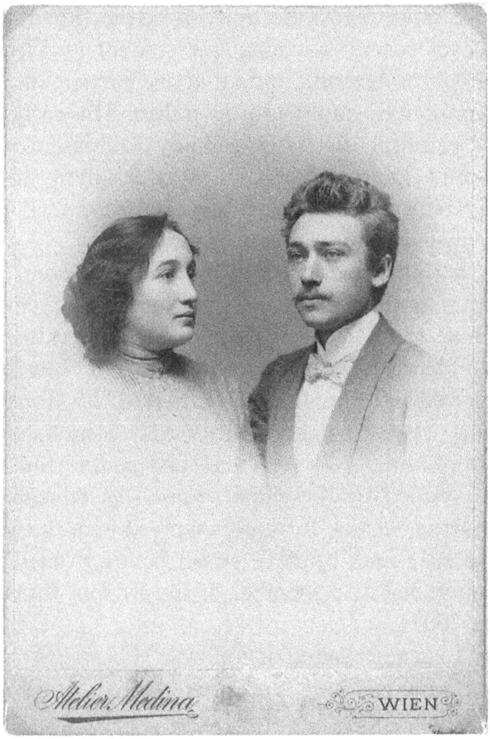

Viktor Tausk with his wife Martha Frisch, c. 1900. Courtesy of Robert Jan Maarten Tausk.

Interestingly, 16 years later, in 1916, Tausk published "Contributions to the psychopathology of everyday life" (Tausk, 1916b/1983a)—not to be confused with a similarly titled posthumous essay first issued in 1934, "Contribution to the psychology of everyday life" (Tausk, 1934/1983a). This latter piece, whose title appears as such in the Spanish edition of Tausk's collected works (Tausk, 1934/1983a, pp. 223–227), is presented under a different heading in the English compilation of his writings, where it is published as "Ibsen the druggist"

(Roazen, 2017a, pp. 221–225). In the final section of the earlier article, "The cult of the ancestors," he recounts the case of "Mr. A.," a man who married a Christian woman unwilling to convert to Judaism and therefore adopted her faith—a passage that is almost certainly autobiographical. At a meeting with his children's tutors, Mr. A. was confronted with antisemitic remarks and decided to conceal his ethnic identity. In one Freudian slip, while dismissing his children to play, he accidentally said, "Go to the garden, Jews (*Juden*)," instead of "children (*Jungen*)" (Tausk, 1916b/1983a).

Kanzer (1972) suggests that Tausk's conversion was likely driven by legal constraints: under Article 64 of the Austrian Civil Code at the time, interfaith marriages were not allowed. Marius Tausk, Viktor Tausk's eldest son, confirmed this, noting that such unions were later subjected to even stricter restrictions by the Christian Social Party (M. Tausk, 1973).

After the wedding, the couple moved to Sarajevo, likely to escape family pressures and financial strain. Tragedy soon followed with the stillbirth of their first child (Roazen, 1980, p. 2). In the aftermath, Viktor resumed his law studies and earned his doctorate in 1902 after completing the three *Rigorosa* exams, despite performing poorly on the first (Eissler, 1983, p. 8). That same year, their eldest son, Marius (1902–1990), was born, followed in 1903 by their second son, Victor Hugo (1903–1969)—the couple's only surviving children (R. J. M. Tausk, personal communication, August 31, 2025).

The naming of their children was deliberate. Martha avoided German names, fearing they might cause trouble in Croatia, while also avoiding Croatian names in case the family returned to Austria (Roazen, 1990). According to Kanzer (1972), Viktor Tausk's rebellious spirit also played a role. The name *Marius* evoked Gaius Marius, the Roman general who triumphed over the aristocracy but was ultimately succeeded by his adoptive son—who met his end in defeat and suicide. The name *Victor Hugo* reflected an admiration for the celebrated French writer who had defied Emperor Napoleon III. As Marius Tausk observes, another factor also influenced the choice: the profound admiration of his paternal grandmother for Hugo's *Le dernier jour d'un condamné* [The last day of a condemned man] (Hugo, 1829), a novel she held in particularly high esteem (M. Tausk, 1973, p. 327).

Whether Viktor Tausk himself ever read the novel remains uncertain, as there is no evidence to confirm it. Yet, in an exercise of free association, one might discern certain resonances between Hugo's work and Tausk's own life—particularly in two respects: first, the condemned man's anguished confrontation with impending death evokes, by analogy, Tausk's clinical interest in the plight of war deserters, many of whom faced execution, an issue he would analyze brilliantly in a 1916 article that will be discussed later in this volume; and second, Tausk's own deeply personal struggle with mortality, culminating in his suicide. Hugo's novel gives voice to a man awaiting execution, capturing the inexorable passage of time, the oscillation between hope and despair, and the suffocating awareness of an approaching end.

Devoid of personal details—the narrator remains nameless, his crime undisclosed—the narrative's force lies in its universality: a human being trapped within an inescapable sentence, suspended between life and death (Hugo, 1829).

Having explored the motivations behind Tausk's marriage on the choice of the names Marius and Victor Hugo for his sons, and my reflections on Hugo's *The last day of a condemned man*—including its potential, if indirect, resonance with the tragic trajectory of Viktor Tausk's own life—I now return to his biography. In 1904, the family relocated to Mostar, where Tausk assumed the position of legal clerk. Here, his work defending marginalized clients, such as a Muslim woman accused of killing her illegitimate child, revealed both his sensitivity to social injustice and his early engagement with human suffering—experiences that would later inform his psychoanalytic thinking (Masotta, 1983). This period, at the intersection of personal responsibility and professional observation, offers a crucial window into the development of his clinical and theoretical sensibilities.

In spring 1905, he qualified for the *stalum agendi*, enabling him to serve as a judge. But instead of continuing his promising legal career, he abandoned it. Freud (1919/1979g) suggested that this was due to deeply personal conflicts, while Viktor himself cited dissatisfaction and discomfort with defending unscrupulous clients. The result was financial instability and a profound professional shift. That same year brought another upheaval: Viktor and Martha's marriage came to an end, and the couple returned to Vienna. Contributing factors included the death of Martha's mother and her yearning to return to Austria (M. Tausk, 1973). In a letter dated March 1, 1906, Viktor confessed to Martha his overwhelming desire for freedom and fear of emotional dependency. He wrote:

> I love only free people, those that are independent of me. For those who depend upon me make me dependent—for this I revenge myself, and then become guilty toward those who did me good. The guilt however eats up the capital, because it bears negative interest of inmensurable dimensions if one wants to pay one's debts [...] The way I am living now is truly the best one for this intention: independent because nobody depends on me, not a slave because not a master.
>
> (Tausk, 1906, as cited in Roazen, 1990, p. 17)

The contents of this letter, in my reading, suggest that Viktor Tausk did not conceive of love as a secure attachment grounded in mutual dependence, where shared intimacy coexists harmoniously with individual autonomy. Rather, his understanding of love seems to rest on a far more polarized and conflict-laden framework, one in which dependency is unconsciously equated with a threat to personal freedom and psychic integrity. Tausk's reflections reveal a profound ambivalence toward relational ties: he refuses to submit to dependence on another, yet resists with equal force the prospect of becoming the object of another's dependence. In his own words, "those who depend upon me make me dependent—for this I revenge myself, and then become guilty towards those who did me good" (Tausk, 1906, as cited in Roazen, 1990, p. 17). This passage opens a window onto a complex psychodynamic process in which dependence is experienced as an invasive demand, mobilizing retaliatory impulses that are swiftly followed by guilt—a guilt that, as he poignantly observes, "eats up the capital," accumulating what he metaphorically describes as "negative interest of incommensurable dimensions."

Such reflections illuminate Tausk's deep-seated difficulty in tolerating asymmetry within libidinal relationships, particularly when these evoke unconscious fantasies of domination and submission. Within this internal drama, the relational dyad seems perpetually suspended between the roles of master and slave—a hierarchical configuration that Tausk explicitly rejects. Against this backdrop, the ideal relational structure he envisions emerges as one of mutual non-dependence: a state he defines as being "independent because nobody depends on me, not a slave because not a master."

Tausk's decision to leave Vienna and relocate to Berlin in 1906 may be read, in this context, not only as a geographical shift but as a defensive maneuver against the perceived entrapments of intimacy. In Berlin, he took up a position as a journalist for the *Berliner Lokalanzeiger*, while his former partner, Martha, remained in Vienna, working as an accountant in her father's publishing house, affiliated with the Social Democratic Party (Eissler, 1983). The spatial and affective distance established through this move reflects a broader psychic strategy aimed at preserving autonomy and mitigating the anxiety elicited by relational dependency. As such, the letter offers a valuable glimpse into the intrapsychic conflicts that shaped Tausk's relational world—a world marked by the unresolved tension between the longing for connection and the fear of enmeshment.

Nonetheless, his relocation to the German capital was far from an untroubled transition. Financial hardship forced Viktor at times to earn money by whistling songs in Berlin bars (Roazen, 1990), a striking image of both material deprivation and psychic dislocation. Despite their separation, Viktor continued to correspond with Martha, who preserved his letters until her death in 1957. These continued communications suggest that, while he may have rejected dependency in principle, affective ties endured in practice—perhaps testifying to the very ambivalence he so poignantly articulated. During his Berlin period, Tausk immersed himself in a remarkably diverse range of intellectual and creative pursuits, reflecting both his versatility and his drive toward symbolic elaboration.

As Lally (2024, p. 104) recounts, Tausk earned a modest living as a journalist and art critic while privately devoting nearly two years to poetry and playwriting during his Berlin period. Among his most significant literary efforts was the draft of "Husein Brko: Bosnische Zigeunergroteske" [Husein Brko: A Bosnian gypsy grotesque], completed around 1906 but not published until 1912. This complex work, which intertwines themes of exile, identity, and tragedy, already reveals Tausk's early engagement with narrative forms that resonated deeply with his existential concerns.

Lally (2024, pp. 259–260) provides a detailed account of this text, noting that "Husein Brko" appeared in four serialized installments in his father's literary review. Drawing on motifs from South Slavic folk ballads while employing the canonical features of the grotesque, Tausk constructs what Lally calls "an oddly anti-oedipal tale." The narrative follows the life of the eponymous bandit Husein—from his supernatural conception to his ignoble death at the hands of his would-be father—while dismantling traditional narrative hierarchies.

It remains uncertain whether "Husein Brko" was conceived from the outset as an anti-oedipal story, but its final form strongly suggests such a reading. Evidence from Tausk's correspondence with Martha around 1906, where he mentions the possibility of publishing the piece in *März*, indicates that the first draft predates his immersion in psychoanalysis. However, his decision to publish the work in 1912, after several years of close engagement with Freud's analytical framework, implies that Freud's teachings inevitably inform its narrative structure and symbolic register (Lally, 2024, p. 259).

While the story shares several striking plot elements with the Oedipus myth, it offers a radically different cultural perspective on hierarchy, destiny, and agency. Unlike Oedipus, whose fate is dictated by divine decree, Husein operates as a "wild actor" within a narrative populated by multiple competing forces. Moreover, the taboos of patricide and incest—central to Sophocles' tragedy—are inverted and deconstructed: in Tausk's tale, they function not as fatal flaws but as grotesque narrative details, stripped of the inevitability that drives the Greek resolution. By adopting the genre of the grotesque, Tausk opens a narrative space in which themes of death, comedy, and existential freedom coexist in tension, revealing an author experimenting with form as much as with meaning.

In addition to "Husein Brko," Tausk produced several existential poems—"Zerstörung" [Destruction], "Das Erbe" [Heritage], "Ziel" [Aim], and "Die Stillen Stunden" [The silent hours]—and created German translations of Serbian folk ballads and literary texts, further reflecting his sustained engagement with themes of identity, belonging, and cultural hybridity (Lally, 2024, p. 104). He also completed a four-act play entitled "Halbdunkel" [Twilight], which appears closely modeled on aspects of his own life, whose protagonist—much like Tausk himself—renounces conventional social status in pursuit of existential meaning. Finally, he drafted a theatrical dialogue between a man of his age and "the sublime Spinoza," a philosophical experiment that underscores his preoccupation with themes of reason, freedom, and destiny.

While a handful of these works appeared in the literary journals *Schaubühne* and *Die Hilfe*, most survive only through preservation in family archives (Lally, 2024, p. 104). Kanzer (1973b) later interpreted this diverse creative production as an attempt by Tausk to impose narrative structure on what he experienced as a fragmented and tumultuous life trajectory.

In parallel with his literary and translation work, Tausk also turned to criticism, reviewing texts such as Gerhart Hauptmann's *Und Pippa tanzt* [And Pippa dances] (Roazen, 1971/1978a; Neumarkt, 1973; Tausk, 1973). Hauptmann (1862–1946), whose full name was Gerhart Johann Robert Hauptmann, was a leading German dramatist and novelist—one of the foremost figures of literary naturalism, though his oeuvre also embraced other stylistic currents—and the recipient of the 1912 Nobel Prize in Literature (Grenville, 2012). Beyond writing, Tausk also cultivated a multifaceted artistic life: he played the violin, painted, composed poetry, and directed theatrical productions. Yet despite this intellectual and creative vitality, Tausk experienced his journalistic career as deeply humiliating—a concession to financial necessity rather than an expression of authentic artistic aspiration.

While this period of intense productivity revealed his polymathic character, it also coincided with a series of romantic involvements that appeared to serve primarily libidinal functions. His numerous affairs with women during these years seem less rooted in emotional intimacy than in sexual gratification—manifestations, perhaps, of his deeply conflicted stance toward relational dependency. This becomes particularly salient, from my perspective, when viewed in the light of Tausk's later notion of *masturbatory coitus*, a concept he elaborated in his 1912 article "On masturbation" (Tausk, 1912/1983a). In this work, Tausk describes masturbatory coitus as a sexual practice focused primarily on the male's discharge, carried out without regard for the woman's pleasure or emotional involvement. Within this configuration, sexual intimacy is transformed into an act of psychic isolation rather than a space of reciprocity—an enactment, at the bodily level, of Tausk's deeper ambivalence toward mutuality, dependence, and emotional connection.

Among these relationships, his affair with dancer Lea Rosen was particularly significant. Although initially passionate, it deteriorated as Tausk's mental health worsened, eventually leading to his admission to a German sanatorium for "mental exhaustion" (M. A. Sperber, 1972; Rodrigué, 1996). Legal proceedings for his divorce cited his affair with Lea, who was largely blamed for the marital breakdown. She later became a patient of Felix Deutsch (1884–1964)—husband of Helene Deutsch, who years afterward served as Viktor Tausk's analyst after Freud declined him—and kept Tausk's letters until her death in Israel in 1972, when the correspondence was ultimately destroyed (Roazen, 1992). These dynamics—of romantic intensity followed by emotional withdrawal, displacement into clinical relationships, and symbolic erasure—mirror Tausk's intrapsychic oscillation between idealization and repudiation, particularly in the context of his relationship with Lea.

Further complexities emerge from accounts of Tausk's professional life. Olga Knopf, one of his students, later accused him of exploiting his position during hypnosis training to seduce female trainees (Eissler, 1983, p. 29). Such conduct—now inevitably viewed through the lens of transference and countertransference—was interpreted by Neumarkt (1977) as evidence of a compulsive pattern possibly concealing repressed homosexuality, against which Tausk adopted a distinctly Don Juan posture. This reading accords with Freud's private theory of Tausk's "psychic impotence," a theme he explored in his correspondence with Sándor Ferenczi. The interplay of erotic compulsion, seduction, and defensive narcissism underscores the central role of sexuality in Tausk's psychic economy—not as a source of genuine intimacy, but as a field of ambivalence, disavowal, and the relentless drive for mastery.

Against this psychological backdrop, Tausk's professional path advanced: in 1911 he began his formative relationship with Helene Deutsch, affectionately known as Hala (Roazen, 1992, p. 9). This meeting was made possible by Joseph Reinhold (1885–1947), a close friend of Deutsch—who had witnessed her wedding and sent her a copy of Freud's *The Interpretation of Dreams* (Freud, 1900/1979a, 1900/1979b)—as well as an intimate friend of Viktor Tausk, whom Reinhold ultimately introduced to her (Roazen, 1990, p. 76). Like Tausk, Reinhold—MD, PhD, a neurologist, philosopher, and psychiatrist trained in Lemberg, Berlin, and Vienna (Nunberg & Federn, 1974, pp. xvi–xvii; Österreichische Akademie der Wissenschaften [ÖAW], 2022)—eventually redirected his career to enter Freud's circle. He completed his hospital training at the Ambulatorium für Nervenkranke, the outpatient neurological department of the University of Vienna, under the distinguished neurologist Lothar Amadeus von Frankl-Hochwart (1862–1914), whose life was cut short by a rapidly progressive brain tumor that claimed him within three months (Triarhou, 2018).

Within the Frankl-Hochwart clinic, Tausk and Deutsch began the collaboration that would lay the foundation for an intellectual and emotional bond soon central to both their lives. Although their professional relationship was grounded in mutual respect, Tausk once remarked that Helene had advanced in her career only by relinquishing her role as wife (Roazen, 1990, p. 76)—a comment that betrays not only the traditional, and arguably sexist, assumptions he held about gender and ambition, but also, in my view, foreshadows the deeper personal and ideological tensions that would later emerge between them.

By late 1907, Tausk's health again declined. Tuberculosis resurfaced alongside severe depression, officially diagnosed as mental exhaustion. He began a rest cure at a German sanatorium in Ahrweiler, trading journalistic articles for free accommodation (Roazen, 1990). In letters to Martha from this period, he expressed a desperate longing for peace, meaningful work, and a loving home.

On October 22, after battling insomnia with medication, Viktor left the clinic and returned to Vienna. There, he discovered Freud through an article and wrote to him. Freud's encouraging reply led Viktor to begin studying psychoanalysis in Vienna—after a restorative trip to Italy (Eissler, 1983, p. 9).

In autumn 1908, he formally entered Freud's circle and started medical studies, supported financially by Freud and the Vienna Psychoanalytic Society. This marked the beginning of his brief but significant career in psychoanalysis. As will be further explored in the following section, psychoanalysis became for Tausk not only an intellectual and clinical vocation but also a deeply personal quest—perhaps a space in which he sought answers to his own existential uncertainties and emotional turmoil. In engaging with this emerging discipline, Tausk may have hoped to resolve his inner conflicts while acquiring the tools to help others similarly afflicted.

Immersion in Psychoanalysis: In Search of Identity and a New Father (1908–1914)

In 1908, after three years of marital separation, Viktor Tausk filed for divorce, which was finalized on October 20 of the same year (R. J. M. Tausk, personal communication, August 31, 2025). Around this same period, he made a decisive move toward becoming a psychoanalyst by enrolling in medical studies at the University of Vienna. His education was financially supported by several prominent members of the psychoanalytic community, including Paul Federn, Josef Karl Friedjung (1871–1946), Eduard Hitschmann (1871–1957), and Ludwig Jekels (1867–1954) (Nunberg & Federn, 1974, p. xvii). Drawing on archival sources and psychoanalytic historiography, Paul Roazen (1990, p. 27) adds to this list Sigmund Freud and Maximilian Steiner (1874–1942), who appears in the *Minutes of the Vienna Psychoanalytic Society* under the variants Maxim Steiner and simply Steiner (Nunberg & Federn, 1962, p. xxxvi). Roazen further notes that four of Freud's Viennese disciples—Hitschmann, Federn, Jekels, and Steiner—jointly awarded Tausk a grant of 4,000 kronen, roughly the equivalent of 800 US dollars at the time.

Further confirmation of Freud's personal involvement can be found in Tausk's own correspondence. In a letter to his former wife dated August 31, 1909, Tausk mentions that Freud had just sent him 150 kronen—although, as he remarked, the sum was insufficient to cover the vacation he had planned. He added, with characteristic irony, that "what is going to come now only Freud and God know." Some might interpret this phrase as a rhetorical flourish—an appeal to fate, with "God and fortune" alone knowing what lies ahead. Yet Tausk, if we take his words literally, places Freud before God in the order of things. Might this suggest that, at that moment, he entrusted his future first to Freud—and only then to God? Be that as it may, during this period Tausk also worked as a journalist. As the saying goes, nothing motivates a human being more than the necessity to survive. Tausk embodied this principle, doing whatever was needed to sustain himself and continue his studies. Despite the support he received, the financial strain of medical training was substantial. Years later, in 1938, his son Marius repaid this educational debt—at the request of Paul Federn—amid the worsening economic conditions in Europe.

Freud, however, graciously declined reimbursement for his contribution, noting that he no longer remembered the amount and, in any case, considered it insignificant. In my view, this gesture reflected a remarkable generosity on Freud's part—effectively writing off a sum he had once lent to support Tausk's medical training. Notably, Marius Tausk would later undergo psychoanalysis free of charge with Hitschmann in 1926, exemplifying the Viennese psychoanalytic community's long-standing ethos of aiding families in psychological or financial distress (Roudinesco & Plon, 1997).

Tausk successfully passed his medical examinations (*Rigorosum*) in March 1911, October 1913, and January 1914, earning his doctorate in June of that year. During his studies, he crossed paths with Edoardo Weiss, a pioneering figure in Italian psychoanalysis who would later found a prominent group that included Marco Levi Bianchini (1875–1961), Nicola Perroti (1897–1970), and Emilio Servadio (1904–1995) (Freud, 1914a/1979d; Sterba, 1985). After being forced to emigrate to the United States, Weiss joined the Menninger Clinic and eventually became a leading member of Franz Alexander's psychoanalytic circle in Chicago (Grotjahn, 1991). Three works by his granddaughter, Ilonka Venier Alexander—a clinical social worker, psychotherapist, and founding scholar of the British Psychoanalytic Council— *The Life and Times of Franz Alexander: From Budapest to California* (Venier Alexander, 2015), *Growing Up Alexander: My Life With a Psychoanalytic Pioneer* (Venier Alexander, 2017), and *The Lost Legacy of Franz Alexander: A Psychoanalytic Pioneer Revisited* (Venier Alexander, 2025) offer a richly documented and deeply reflective account of the personal and professional trajectory of Franz Alexander (1891–1964), one of the most innovative and influential figures in the history of psychoanalysis.

Well before his eventual emigration to the United States, Weiss recalled that he and Tausk had attended the same medical courses and collaborated at the neurological clinic of Frankl-Hochwart, a prominent opponent of Freud and psychoanalysis who frequently ridiculed both. For his specialization in psychiatry and neurology, Tausk trained under Julius von Wagner-Jauregg (1857–1940), a former classmate of Freud and Nobel Prize laureate in medicine for his development of malariotherapy in the treatment of general paresis (Hamilton, 1991).

At that time, few psychiatrists were seriously engaged with psychoanalysis. Among them was the Swiss psychiatrist Ludwig Binswanger (1881–1966), owner of the Bellevue Sanatorium in Kreuzlingen on Lake Constance, who attended—*as a guest*—a session of the Vienna Psychoanalytic Society on January 19, 1910 (Nunberg & Federn, 1967, p. 394). He would later remark on how isolated psychoanalytic inquiry still was within psychiatric circles. Yet, interest among physicians from other medical disciplines was beginning to grow. That same year, at a medical congress held in Baden-Baden, Alfred Erich Hoche (1865–1943), professor of psychiatry at the University of Freiburg im Breisgau, delivered a provocative lecture titled "A psychic epidemic among physicians," in which he sharply denounced psychoanalysis and its expanding influence (Freud, 1914a/1979d).

According to Weiss (1991, p. 9), his friendship with Tausk began during their time at the School of Medicine and lasted until 1914, when both completed their studies. Apart from a brief reunion during World War I, their close contact was limited to this academic period. During those years, they frequently discussed theoretical and technical aspects of psychoanalysis, as well as personal matters related to Freud and other members of the psychoanalytic circle.

Tausk regularly attended the Wednesday meetings of the Vienna Psychoanalytic Society and was listed as one of its 23 members in a document dated October 1909. This record was presented at the opening session of the Society's eighth year, held on October 12, 1909, at the Hotel Residenz, where Tausk was initially noted as a guest (Nunberg & Federn, 1967, p. 278). He was formally nominated as a full member on October 27 (Nunberg & Federn, 1967, p. 282) and officially confirmed on November 3 (Nunberg & Federn, 1967, p. 290).

Viktor Tausk's first paper to the Vienna Psychoanalytic Society, entitled "Theory of knowledge and psychoanalysis," was presented on November 24, 1909, before an audience that included many of the leading figures of early psychoanalysis: Sigmund Freud, Alfred Adler (1870–1937), Paul Federn, Josef Karl Friedjung, Carl Furtmüller (1880–1951), Max Graf (1873–1958), Eduard Hitschmann, Ludwig Jekels, and Albert Joachim (1877–?), about whom—unlike nearly all other members of the Society—almost nothing is known beyond a few scattered facts: that he was born on January 7, 1877, in Aujezd, Moravia; that he completed his *Matura* in Brünn and earned his medical degree in 1903 (Gelfand & Kerr, 2013, p. 73); and that he later served as director of a sanatorium in Rekawinkel, then regarded as one of the finest private institutions for mental patients near Vienna (Nunberg & Federn, 1962, p. xxxv). The audience also included Otto Rank (1884–1939), Rudolf Reitler (1865–1917), and Isidor Isaak Sadger (1867–1942; hereafter referred to simply as Isidor Sadger or Sadger). Before mentioning the other attendees, a brief note may be of interest to attentive readers. The works by Sadger cited in this book (see the final "References" section) appear under the initial J. rather than I.—a convention reflecting early twentieth-century German typographical practice, in which the letters *I* and *J* were often used interchangeably in proper names. This peculiarity is also mirrored in the records of the four-volume *Minutes*, where, beginning with Vol. 3, Sadger is listed as Dr. J. Sadger, whereas in the earlier volumes he appears simply as Dr. Sadger. With this clarification, alongside Rank, Reitler, and Sadger, the meeting was also attended by Maxim Steiner, Wilhelm Stekel (1868–1940), and Fritz

Wittels (1880–1950). As the editors of the *Minutes* observe in a footnote, "the topic is difficult; a reader who is not well versed in philosophy may well find it difficult to understand," adding that Rank's summary of the lecture was somewhat cursory and may have contributed to gaps in the transcript (Nunberg & Federn, 1967, p. 332).

Beginning his presentation, Tausk gave a concise overview of the history of epistemology and its fundamental problems. He insisted on the necessity of distinguishing between two different subjects: the function of perception and the function of the instincts, including affects and drives. The theory of knowledge, he argued, concerns the investigation of functional processes. He traced the lineage of epistemological thought on perception in a narrowly defined sense, from Aristotle (384–322 BCE) through Baruch Spinoza (1632–1677) to David Hume (1711–1776), who represents the true beginning of modern epistemology. Hume introduced the psychological challenge of explaining causality; however, according to Tausk, Hume was only partially correct, as he lacked a psychology of perception—an omission that Immanuel Kant (1724–1804) later addressed. In this respect, Kant proposed that relations such as time, space, causality, quality, and quantity exist only within the mind. These are *a priori* conditions shaping how we organize and interpret objects and events. This framework marked the first psychology of knowledge, later systematized by Kant into a refined yet, in Tausk's view, diluted structure. Freud's discoveries, by contrast, redirected attention to the primacy of affective experience. Tausk argued that the fundamental error of philosophers such as Hume, Kant, and Arthur Schopenhauer (1788–1860) was their attempt to impose the harmonious logic of pure thought upon beings who are, by nature, imperfect and conflict-ridden. For Tausk, conflict is not an anomaly in human life but a prerequisite for existence. In support of this view, he drew heavily on Freud's psychological laws, emphasizing in particular the dynamics of repression and anxiety. Repression furnishes the symbolic, sublimated material that underlies epistemological theories, while anxiety acts as their psychic driving force. Consciousness and instinctual life thus become the core subjects of the theory of knowledge, with consciousness functioning to recognize the unconscious. In relation to this, the editors of the *Minutes* clarify in a footnote that this definition should not be conflated with Freud's own concept of consciousness, which he conceived as an organ for perceiving both external events and internal processes—including preconscious and unconscious ideas, feelings, and sensations (Nunberg & Federn, 1967, p. 331). Freud further maintained that consciousness develops through the differentiation of feelings, conditioned by environmental challenges, and emerges as a survival mechanism conferring an adaptive advantage over individuals governed solely by instinctual satisfaction.

The relationship between consciousness and the unconscious first emerged through disturbances in function, which prompted investigations into the laws governing mental functioning. A disturbed function is understood as one in the process of adaptation. Regarding the origin of consciousness in terms of environmental conditions, Tausk posited that the weakest individuals of a particular quality are the first to develop consciousness, leading to the notion that civilization is "a civilization of the weak." This view was later contested by Friedjung, who argued instead that civilization is "always a civilization of the strong." From my perspective, this disagreement evokes Nietzschean undercurrents—above all, the figure of the *Übermensch* and the interplay of Apollonian and Dionysian forces so central to his thought. I return to these ideas briefly—not as a philosophical detour, but because they illuminate the intellectual spirit in which this scientific meeting unfolded. The *Übermensch*, for Nietzsche, represents the individual who transcends conformity to create and live by self-fashioned values—a stark contrast to the "last man," who seeks comfort and evades conflict. This ideal reflects a transformation of instinct into creative, life-affirming energy. Similarly, Nietzsche's polarity between Apollonian order and Dionysian impulse mirrors the psychoanalytic tension between ego organization and instinctual drive. In this sense, the *Übermensch* may be viewed as a symbolic figure of sublimation—a psyche that has overcome repression by converting drive energy into culturally generative expression.

Returning to Tausk's presentation, while his views diverged in certain respects from those of other participants, he was fully aware of, and openly acknowledged, the provisional nature of his exposition. Yet he remained convinced that he had demonstrated something essential: that Freud's psychological laws could be meaningfully extended into the domain of epistemological inquiry. He criticized the term "*metapsychology*" and suggested that "*transcendental psychology*" would be more appropriate, as it better conveys the idea of a psychology concerned with revealing unconditional functions. The editors of the *Minutes*, however, did not share this terminological preference and observed that, in keeping with their editorial principles, they refrained from offering explicit commentary—even when they perceived Tausk to diverge from Freud's theoretical positions (Nunberg & Federn, 1967, p. 332).

At the conclusion of the session, Freud offered several critiques, advising Tausk to present his ideas in less abstract terms and to elaborate further in future presentations, particularly regarding material not yet included (Nunberg & Federn, 1967, p. 335). During that same meeting of November 24, 1909, an additional episode occurred—absent from the official *Minutes of the Vienna Psychoanalytic Society*—that has come down to us solely through Wilhelm Stekel's own written testimony. In his intimate and personal memoir, *The Autobiography of Wilhelm Stekel: The Life Story of a Pioneer Psychoanalyst* (Gutheil, 1950), specifically in Chapter 5—titled "The break with Freud" (pp. 127–145)—Stekel, as will be discussed shortly, offered his own account of the incident with Tausk on that occasion.

According to Stekel's recollection, although Tausk began his presentation with impressive self-assurance, midway through he lost his train of thought and was ultimately unable to finish (Gutheil, 1950, p. 133). Stekel described the moment as awkward for all present. Seeking to salvage the situation, he stepped in and continued the lecture extemporaneously. Perhaps for this reason, Stekel speculated, Tausk never forgave him. As further evidence of the unresolved tension, Stekel later recalled that, at the very next opportunity, Tausk subjected his new book to sharp criticism, dwelling at length on the grammatical errors in its preface. Tausk's criticisms of Stekel's work, as will be discussed shortly, took place during the meeting of November 2, 1910—a session in which Stekel, in his own defense, explained that he typically wrote in haste (Gutheil, 1950, p. 133).

The book in question was *Die Sprache des Traumes. Eine Darstellung der Symbolik und Deutung des Traumes in ihren Beziehungen zur kranken und gesunden Seele für Ärzte und Psychologen* [The language of dreams. A presentation for physicians and psychologists of the interpretation and symbolism of the dream in its relation to both the sick and healthy mind] (Stekel, 1911). That same year, the book reached the psychoanalytic community through a review by Ernest Jones published in *The Journal of Abnormal Psychology* (Jones, 1911). Thanks to the meticulous research of Stekel's scholar Francis Clark-Lowes, we also know that, 11 years later, an English translation of only the first part appeared under the title *Sex and Dreams: The Language of Dreams* (Stekel, 1922), translated by Van Teslaar (Clark-Lowes, 2010, p. 257). Nearly two decades later, another English edition was released under the title *The Interpretation of Dreams* (Stekel, 1943). Yet, despite its 1911 publication date, Stekel had already referred to the book during the scientific meeting of the Vienna Psychoanalytic Society held on November 2, 1910, where, as mentioned earlier, Tausk sharply criticized aspects of the forthcoming volume. On that occasion, as recorded in the *Minutes*, Stekel presented his paper "The choice of a profession and neurosis"—a topic whose discussion extended into the following session on November 9, 1910 (Nunberg & Federn, 1974). In the November 2 session, Stekel observed that death plays a far greater role in dreams than had previously been assumed, adding that in his forthcoming book—which we now know to be the 1911 volume—he had cataloged a considerable number of these death symbols (Nunberg & Federn, 1974, p. 38).

It is significant, however, that the official *Minutes* of the November 2, 1910, meeting contain no record of Tausk's specific critique of Stekel's preface. Nor do they support the claim, sometimes repeated, that Tausk rejected the entire book rather than the preface alone (Eissler, 1971, p. 58). Eissler's assertion predates the publication of the *Minutes* volume covering that session, which appeared only in 1974. The explanation lies in Eissler's own admission, in the preface to his 1971 work, *Talent and Genius* (p. xii), that he had been granted permission by the editors of the *Minutes*, Herman Nunberg and Ernst Federn, to consult unpublished portions of the Society's records that contained references to Tausk.

Stekel's autobiographical account adds still further texture to the November 2, 1910, meeting. He wrote that subsequent speakers also disparaged his work—many focusing exclusively on the preface. Expecting Freud to offer at least some words in his defense, Stekel was disappointed to find that even Freud remained silent. The only exception, he noted, was Adler, who at that time still counted himself among Stekel's friends (Gutheil, 1950, p. 133).

If these episodes indeed marked the origins of the discord between Tausk and Stekel, the following years did little to ease their mutual animosity. Its persistence is evident in Jones's (1955) later remarks in the second volume of his Freud biography, where he explicitly referred to the personal hostility between the two men (p. 136). In tracing its roots, however, Jones attributed Tausk's dislike of Stekel to a rather vague cause and incorrectly placed the conflict in 1912—an interpretation that, as I have already established, lacks any factual basis.

Although I will return to this point in greater detail later in this book, it is important to note here that Jones appears to have been unaware of what transpired during the scientific meetings held on November 24, 1909, and November 2, 1910. From my perspective, this omission was not intentional but can likely be explained by two factors. First, the second and third volumes of the *Minutes of the Vienna Psychoanalytic Society*—covering 1908–1910 (Vol. 2) and 1910–1911 (Vol. 3)—were not published until 1967 and 1974, respectively (Nunberg & Federn, 1967, 1974), appearing 12 and 19 years after the release of Jones's second volume. It is, therefore, highly probable that Jones was simply unaware of their contents. Second, unlike Eissler, Jones seems not to have consulted Stekel's autobiography (Gutheil, 1950), published five years before his own work (Jones, 1955), in which Stekel offered a candid and detailed account of the origins and intensity of his conflict with Tausk.

Beyond these contentious events, Tausk remained an active and engaged participant in the scientific meetings of the Vienna Psychoanalytic Society. One particularly striking intervention occurred on April 6, 1910, shortly after the tense Nuremberg Congress, where frictions had intensified between the Viennese group, led by Adler, and other factions. Although Tausk had not attended the congress himself, he perceptively remarked that he had sensed something profoundly unsettling had occurred. With characteristic irony, he observed that no soil was more fertile for the growth of Freud's ideas than Vienna—precisely because it was "sick" soil.

This aphoristic observation, while outwardly affirming loyalty to the Viennese circle, carried an unmistakable undertone: an acute recognition of the morbid currents animating the Society's internal life. In retrospect, it reads as a deftly veiled critique of Adler, whose rising influence within the group was already a source of contention. The comment thus functioned on two levels—outward solidarity with Freud's camp, and a subtle act of boundary-setting *vis-à-vis* the ideological direction Adler was steering.

Such moments reveal a facet of Tausk often overshadowed by accounts of his later conflicts: his ability to diagnose, with clinical precision, the latent tensions structuring psychoanalytic politics. This capacity to read the unspoken dynamics at play would resurface repeatedly in the years to follow, shaping not only his relationships with individual colleagues, but also his evolving theoretical contributions. Far from being a passive observer of Freud's inner circle, Tausk was a shrewd interlocutor—one who navigated its rivalries with a blend of wit, skepticism, and strategic alignment.

This acuity proved particularly valuable in the turbulent months that followed. In this fraught climate, and in the wake of the Society's internal restructuring—Freud's bid to forestall further fragmentation through the creation of the International Psychoanalytical Association (IPA) and the appointment of Carl Gustav Jung (1875–1961) as its first president—Adler nevertheless retained his position as head of the Viennese group. Only days later, on April 20, 1910, a scientific session was held in which David Ernst Oppenheim (1881–1943) presented a critical review of an essay by Abraham Adolf Baer (1834–1908), a German physician and leading figure of the social-hygiene movement. The essay, *Der Selbstmord im kindlichen Lebensalter* [Suicide in childhood] (Baer, 1901), explored the unsettling phenomenon of self-destruction in children (Nunberg & Federn, 1967, p. 481). The debate resumed on April 27 in a follow-up meeting devoted to suicide more broadly, during which Tausk offered a penetrating intervention that revealed both his clinical acuity and his wide theoretical reach.

Addressing the problem of suicidal behavior in children, Tausk highlighted the central role of an intense, often unconscious, sense of guilt. Importantly, he drew a distinction between two separate dimensions of the problem: first, the question of the *meaning* of suicide; and second, the question of the *psychic mechanisms* underlying it. These two questions, he argued, may point to fundamentally distinct avenues of inquiry—one interpretive, the other metapsychological—both of which warranted careful analytic exploration (Nunberg & Federn, 1967, pp. 501–502).

Regarding the first, Tausk referred to Schopenhauer's view that "life is a stance," and from this standpoint, suicide represents an individual's illogical action *kat' exochén*—that is, *the most illogical act par excellence*, a radical denial of life's foundational affirmation. He then sought to translate this existential stance into biological terms, thereby giving it psychological meaning as well.

Tausk proceeded to explore in depth the concept of the sense of guilt, which he identified as the psychological ground upon which any internal conflict leading to suicide must rest. Guilt, he argued, ultimately stems from civilization's demands, which compel individuals either to sublimate or repress instinctual drives. The father appears as the figure who embodies and enforces this demand—often with greater severity the more he himself has failed to meet it. The child perceives this failure and unconsciously criticizes the father, thus generating a fundamental psychic conflict. While the precise psychic mechanisms that transform this negation into a positive drive toward suicide remain unspecified in this discussion, Tausk asserted with certainty that sexual elements are involved.

He concluded by recalling several suicides among teachers during his own school years, noting that, in many cases, teachers may inadvertently become the immediate triggers for suicide precisely because they are not allowed to acknowledge that children are "loaded" with sexuality. Although society has changed considerably since Tausk spoke these words in 1910, the tragedy of youth suicide persists. Even today, many children take their own lives as a result of bullying, abuse, or other forms of violence. In my view, psychoanalysis, much as it did then, still has a crucial role to play in uncovering the unconscious meanings behind such acts and in offering insights that could help prevent them.

Allow me a brief aside—though I will return to this topic in greater depth later. It is profoundly poignant that Tausk, despite the penetrating analyses of suicide he offered during the Vienna Psychoanalytic Society's meeting of April 27, 1910—a session devoted to the general discussion of suicide, following the debate a week earlier on April 20 of Baer's *Suicide in childhood*—was ultimately unable to avert his own death nine years later, in 1919, at the age of 40. In that April 27 meeting, as I have seen, he described suicide as an illogical act *kat' exochén*—a formulation that, when read against the arc of his life, acquires a quiet, almost unbearable poignancy.

Less than a month later, on May 18, 1910, following Stekel's presentation on "The feeling of strangeness in dream and in life," Tausk contributed a characteristically incisive intervention to the discussion—one that revealed both his capacity for theoretical nuance and his sensitivity to the subtleties of human experience. He referred to Freud's example of a familiar word that suddenly loses its meaning, interpreting this phenomenon as a divestment of the word's affective charge within the sentence—that is, within the complex. Drawing on his own experience, Tausk suggested that the feeling of estrangement often arises alongside a deep sense of guilt (Nunberg & Federn, 1967, pp. 539–540). He went so far as to propose that this emotional state might signify an unbearable self-recognition: "If I recognize myself, then I must kill myself." In this light, he interpreted Adler's case of the schoolboy as fitting within this category. As a counterpart to such existential despair, Tausk cited the often-quoted notion that society itself is nothing but a comedy—arguing that even this cynical view masks a latent sense of guilt.

In his psychological analysis of estrangement, Tausk emphasized the need to distinguish whether the perceived strangeness stems from general unrecognizability or from a specific change in the object—such as an addition or subtraction. Each of these variations, he argued, carries its own meaning. Ultimately, Tausk posited that experiences of depersonalization and self-estrangement are closely linked to unconscious guilt and may even culminate in suicidal ideation.

His stark formulation—"If I recognize myself, then I must kill myself" (Nunberg & Federn, 1967, p. 540)—demonstrates his characteristic use of introspection to illuminate clinical problems. In hindsight, it also foreshadows the internal conflicts that would tragically lead to his own death.

The theme of suicide, tragically, did not end with Viktor. His sister, Ilka—better known to family and friends as Jelka—ended her life on August 17, 1938, together with her husband, Ernst Maximilian Gans, and his twin brother, Camillo, in the aftermath of the Nazi invasion. Born in 1880, Jelka worked as a teacher and midwife. She had previously been married to a Yugoslav physician, Bodo (R. J. M. Tausk, personal communication, August 31, 2025), but following an unhappy marriage—and encouraged by Viktor—she divorced. On September 7, 1912, she married Ernst, an Austrian philologist and teacher of Latin and Greek, who was also one of Viktor's close friends. He shared a home with Camillo, a respected tax lawyer, and together they provided Jelka with a sense of stability and happiness she had not known before. On several occasions, Viktor visited their home, often accompanied by a female companion, and among these, Jelka was reportedly especially fond of Ilse Zimmermann (Roazen, 1990, p. 109).

By 1912, a new romantic entanglement would profoundly shape Viktor Tausk's life. That year, and into the next, he became involved in a passionate affair with Lou Andreas-Salomé (1861–1937), a charismatic and influential figure within the early psychoanalytic community. At 51, she was already renowned for her relationships with Friedrich Nietzsche (1844–1900), Rainer Maria Rilke (1875–1926), and other leading intellectuals—a testament to her keen mind and capacity for profound spiritual and intellectual connection. Since 1887, she had been married to Friedrich Carl Andreas (1846–1930), an orientalist philologist and polyglot whose scholarship spanned the history of languages, civilizations, philosophy, and natural history (Farridnejad, 2016). Yet her marriage did not preclude her from forming a deep emotional bond with Tausk. Their relationship created a complex triangle between Lou, Tausk, and Freud—a pattern that would repeat when Tausk later underwent analysis with Helene Deutsch, who was herself in analysis with Freud. In both cases, these arrangements allowed Freud to maintain a degree of control over the unpredictable Tausk by receiving indirect insights through trusted female confidants.

Freud employed a similar strategy through Sándor Ferenczi (1873–1933), one of his most prominent disciples. In a letter dated April 12, 1913, Ferenczi informed Freud that he had attempted to extract information about Tausk from Lou, promising to share the limited details he had gathered when they next met in Vienna (Falzeder et al., 1994, p. 478).

Freud's and Tausk's fascination with Lou Andreas-Salomé stemmed not only from her undeniable beauty but, more significantly, from her extraordinary intellect. Her brilliance was expressed through a prolific and nuanced body of work: over 20 books and more than a hundred essays, articles, and critical reflections. To these achievements must be added her fiercely independent spirit, which intensified her personal magnetism (Peters, 1962/1995), as well as her uncanny ability to awaken the creative faculties of the men who loved her—while she herself often maintained a deliberate emotional distance (Roazen, 1971/1978a, 1990).

Given the breadth of her intellectual production and the singularity of her presence, it seems unlikely that Lou sought proximity to influential men—Freud, Nietzsche, Rilke, or Tausk—in a bid for reflected glory. Quite the contrary: her legacy suggests a woman whose brilliance stood on its own terms. In this regard, Eissler (1971) offers a particularly compelling observation. Reflecting on Andreas-Salomé's pattern of attachment, he writes:

> The fact that so many of those to whom she was close were not known, or little known, or rejected, but later rose to extraordinary fame—that very fact is proof of her uncanny intuition and knowledge about man, which served her in her unfailing recognition of true values. That this woman, whose mind was equal to that of the greatest of her times, found gratification and pleasure mainly in the company of extraordinary minds was not a result of snobbishness, or arrogance, or of a rage for "name-dropping," but rather a necessity—unless one thinks that she should have been content with the boredom generated by mediocrities.
>
> (p. 44)

This assessment aptly captures the paradox at the heart of Lou Andreas-Salomé's life and work: she was drawn to exceptional minds not out of vanity, but because of an intellectual and emotional vitality that could only be nourished by genuine brilliance. Her presence in the lives of these men was not parasitic but catalytic—never simply a muse, she was a thinker in her own right, a participant in, rather than a shadow of, the cultural and psychological revolutions that defined her era.

This portrait of Lou Andreas-Salomé as a woman of intellectual independence and emotional discernment finds a complementary, if more polemical, counterpart in the reflections of Emilio Rodrigué. While Eissler (1971) emphasized her intuitive depth and the authenticity of her affinities, Rodrigué (1996) approaches her from a more psychologically dramatized angle—one that foregrounds not only her charisma but also the dynamics of desire and sublimation that marked her relationships with men of genius.

According to Rodrigué (1996), Lou—evocatively dubbed "the sorceress of Hainberg" and "Lady of the triangles"—turned her attention to Tausk after her unsuccessful attempt to win Freud as a lover. At the time, Tausk was 34, while Lou was 51, a difference that highlights the encounter between a younger analyst and a mature, intellectually seasoned figure. In Rodrigué's metaphorical phrasing, it was Tausk who came to occupy one of the most prominent places in "Freud's henhouse." For her part, Lou would later describe him as the most distinguished among Freud's disciples.

Rodrigué's interpretation, while more speculative in tone, does not necessarily contradict Eissler's. Rather, it introduces an additional layer of complexity to Andreas-Salomé's psycho-emotional universe: one in which unfulfilled desire, admiration, and symbolic substitution may have intersected. His view invites us to consider that Lou's bonds were not only shaped by intellectual affinities or aesthetic appreciation, but also by deeper, more ambiguous undercurrents of longing and relational displacement—forces that psychoanalysis itself teaches us to acknowledge.

Far from being a one-sided dynamic of admiration or symbolic substitution, the relationship between Lou Andreas-Salomé and Tausk unfolded as an active exchange—intellectual, clinical, and affective. While Lou offered Tausk a space of reflection and emotional resonance, he in turn facilitated her engagement with the practical dimensions of clinical work. It was Tausk who introduced her to the neurological clinic of Frankl-Hochwart, enabling her to observe psychiatric cases firsthand—a formative experience that no doubt deepened her understanding of psychopathology and its embodied expressions.

Their shared interests extended beyond the scientific. Tausk entrusted Lou with several Serbian ballads he had translated, revealing a more poetic dimension of his sensibility. On several occasions, she even accompanied him on visits to his children—gestures that signal a bond not merely intellectual, but grounded in the everyday realities of care and relational presence.

One particularly striking episode, originally recorded by Lou Andreas-Salomé in her *Der Schule bei Freud. Tagebuch eines Jahres, 1912–1913* [In Freud's school: Diary of a year, 1912–1913] (Andreas-Salomé, 1958/1984), vividly illustrates the spirit of clinical experimentation that characterized Tausk's work at the Frankl-Hochwart clinic. Since this diary was published posthumously in 1958, it is important—before discussing its content—to clarify an issue of terminology that may otherwise cause confusion. The same work was later released in English under a different title, *The Freud Journal of Lou Andreas-Salomé* (1958/1984). To ensure clarity and consistency, in what follows I will refer to this text exclusively as *The Freud Journal.*

In this autobiographical account, Lou documents an especially provocative and ethically complex experiment conducted by Tausk: he applied galvanic stimulation to the genital area of a woman who had undergone an oophorectomy, seeking to determine whether the operation had impaired her orgasmic response. That Lou either witnessed or meticulously recorded this episode underscores not only her close proximity to Tausk's professional life but also her exposure to the more fraught and exploratory dimensions of early psychosexual research.

Regarding Lou's relationship with Freud, she traced the beginning of their friendship to the autumn of 1911, in the wake of the Third International Psychoanalytic Congress held in Weimar, Germany, on September 21–22 of that year. She recounts this in her intimate and evocative autobiographical work *Lebensrückblick: Grundriss einiger Lebenserinnerungen* [Looking back:

A sketch of some life memories] (Andreas-Salomé, 1951/1988), published in English as *Looking Back: Memoirs.* However, other evidence suggests that their first encounter may have taken place 16 years earlier, in 1895. This possibility is raised in the prologue to her other autobiographical work, *The Freud Journal* (Andreas-Salomé, 1958/1984), written in 1957 by Ernst Pfeiffer (1893–1986), Lou's literary executor, who recalls Lucia Morawitz's remark that she once had to interrupt a conversation with Andreas-Salomé, who was due to meet Freud shortly thereafter (Pfeiffer, 1958/1984). Supporting this view, González (1997) observes that, in 1895—at the encouragement of Arthur Schnitzler (1862–1931), later associated with the literary circle *Young Vienna*—Lou paid a brief visit to Freud.

Although Lou herself does not mention this encounter in her writings, circumstantial evidence lends it plausibility. Among her surviving papers are several psychiatric manuscripts from that period, revealing an early and distinctly clinical interest in psychopathological themes. Pfeiffer suggests that Lou's early interest may have been ignited by her exposure to *Studies on Hysteria* (Breuer & Freud, 1893–1895/1980)—a seminal work of which no copy was found among her possessions, perhaps lost during the purges of the Nazi era (Andreas-Salomé, 1958/1984). Moreover, during the winter of 1884–1885, Lou visited her brother Eugène in Vienna, where he was training under Hermann Nothnagel (1841–1905), a distinguished internist at the University of Vienna.

Nevertheless, Lou's biographer Peters (1962/1995) maintains that her first documented encounter with Freud took place at the Weimar Congress, facilitated by Poul Carl Bjerre (1876–1964), a Swedish psychiatrist with whom she was then romantically involved. Lou had met Bjerre in the salon of the Swedish writer Ellen Key (1849–1926), both a distant relative of his and a close friend and admirer of Rainer Maria Rilke—who, in time, would become Lou's lover. By the 1930s, Bjerre would distance himself from Freudian theory and, under Jung's influence, emerge as a leading figure within the General Medical Society for Psychotherapy (Freud & Jung, 1974/1978).

Peters (1962/1995) also suggests that Lou's interest in psychoanalysis was nurtured by her earlier relationship with Friedrich Nietzsche, who taught her that human behavior is driven more by unconscious instincts than by rational thought. In her autobiographical notes (Andreas-Salomé, 1958/1984), Lou credits her initial curiosity about psychoanalysis to the writings of Hermann Swoboda (1873–1963), a psychology professor at the University of Vienna. Disenchanted with the prevailing experimental psychology of his time, Swoboda proposed that the unconscious psyche operated in recurrent cycles, analogous to biological rhythms—a notion he elaborated in his 1904 essay *Die Perioden des menschlichen Organismus in ihrer psychologischen und biologischen Bedeutung* [The periods of the human organism in their psychological and biological significance] (Swoboda, 1904). These notions were, in essence, an extension of the earlier speculations on biological periodicity advanced by the German otolaryngologist Wilhelm Fließ (1858–1928), whose close friendship and theoretical collaboration with Freud are well known. Freud had already engaged with Fließ's ideas—critically and with notable reserve—in *The Interpretation of Dreams* (Freud, 1900/1979a, 1900/1979b).

From another vantage point—and only a few months before the Third International Psychoanalytic Congress convened in Weimar at the end of September 1911—Viktor Tausk delivered his paper "A contribution to the psychology of masochism" at a scientific meeting on May 10 of that year. He prefaced his remarks by noting that they drew on a single case, acknowledging the limitations of his observations while hinting at the broader implications for understanding masochistic phenomena.

To begin with, Tausk described the patient's character as it appeared externally: someone who pretended to be less intelligent than he actually was—a man who deliberately concealed his knowledge. In truth, he had led a consciously active sexual life since the age of 5 and had learned to hide this fact. He had discharged his entire sexuality through masochistic fantasies and, up until the beginning of treatment, had never engaged in sexual intercourse. It later became clear that he also suffered from a diffuse obsessive neurosis that had somewhat delayed his development. At this point, Tausk emphasized the importance of distinguishing between symptoms arising from neurosis and those related to perversion. In the context of his presentation, he would focus solely on the latter. A central figure in both the patient's neurosis and his masochistic fantasies was the mother. Until he was aged 9, there had been a strong bond between them. However, when she became attracted to his tutor, her attitude changed drastically—she began to mistreat the child, beating him, suspecting him, and showing clear hostility. The boy was devastated and experienced a profound conflict that lasted around three years, after which he turned completely away from his mother. At the time, Tausk reported, the patient genuinely hated her. Tausk also observed that he shifted his affections to his father, whom he had previously both feared and disliked.

This contrast in emotional orientation toward the mother is also reflected in the content of the patient's masochistic fantasies: elegant women in these fantasies never actively do anything to him or make physical contact. In a brief footnote, the editors of the *Minutes* remarked that this passage is not entirely clear (Nunberg & Federn, 1974, p. 252). One might assume, Tausk continued, that the mother's behavior directly caused the masochism—but this was not the case. Rather, she became the material that the fantasy structure later employed. Tausk then broadened the discussion to include other significant findings from the analysis—matters of particular relevance to psychoanalytic theory. These included early childhood sexual behavior: mutual genital exhibition between children, masturbation at age 6, and displays of the buttocks. Among the patient's infantile sexual theories were the beliefs that children are born through the anus, and that his sister once had a penis, which was later cut off. In the patient's mind, the penis and buttocks were not clearly distinguished; for example, he would insert irritating objects into the urethra, analogously to enemas. The patient's masochistic fantasies began around age 6—well before the shift in his mother's behavior. Tausk referred to the "limits set by amnesia" (*Amnesiengrenze*), which in this case extended back to the sixth year of life and appeared to be linked to a serious illness the patient had suffered. His early fantasies were extremely violent: he imagined being taken into the kitchen, where his abdomen was cut open, his intestines removed, and he died in unbearable pain. These fantasies also included the cutting off of buttocks, thighs, and the head—though the genitals remained untouched until puberty. Over time, the patient's fantasies grew more complex and psychologically sophisticated. He imagined elaborate scenes involving numerous characters drawn from real life.

Until puberty, the patient in Tausk's case consistently imagined himself in his masochistic fantasies to be the same age he was in reality. However, once he reached the age of 20, he continued to portray himself in those fantasies as an adolescent—an observation that, according to Tausk, supports Freud's hypothesis that perversion constitutes a developmental arrest.

Tausk then turns to an analysis of the origins and composition of the fantasy material itself. He highlights how certain scenes and characters were shaped by the patient's lived experience, and illustrates—through the patient's own explanations—how even a seemingly minor compromise formation can be deconstructed. For instance, the patient introduces external agents, such as figures who force him to undress, to preserve his own sense of innocence. This displacement of guilt is tightly bound to a castration fantasy that emerged during puberty, which was itself catalyzed by a rumor about an army officer allegedly punished by castration.

A third perspective on the patient's guilt—a perspective underscoring the intrinsic link between sadism and masochism—is revealed in the way the patient responds to repressed rage: he channels it into masochistic fantasies. From age 14, he reported fantasizing nightly and experiencing at least one nocturnal emission each night. He masturbated regularly until the age of 17, when fear instilled by a book led him to achieve ejaculation without physical stimulation.

Tausk next engages with the core question: How can a person derive sexual pleasure from suffering or mistreatment? He proposes two explanatory avenues. First, the patient habitually bit his lips and hands in moments of intense anger, a behavior Tausk interprets as a pathological form of abreaction—an attempt to discharge abnormal sadistic impulses. This might give the impression that pain itself becomes a source of pleasure. In the fantasies, the infliction of pain by women serves as a symbolic punishment—an externalization of guilt. The patient was consciously aware of his sexual feelings toward his mother and struggled to repress them. Second, another explanatory path emerged through technical analysis. Here, feelings of inferiority—central to Adlerian theory—coincided with a range of anal-erotic symptoms. These included extended and intricate patterns of forepleasure centered on anal sensations. In recent attempts at intercourse, the patient did not experience penile erection, and described coitus as emotionally insignificant. He associated the sexual act with the image of an "upright anus," which evoked fantasies of passive pederasty. His inability to perceive penile sensation, described by Tausk as a form of hysterical anesthesia, symbolically declared: "there shall be no penis here."

Tausk infers that in this patient, the anus had become the erotogenic zone, replacing the vagina. All early masochistic fantasies were fundamentally anal; in fact, the patient did not distinguish between buttocks and penis. His castration fantasy progressed to the point where he imagined a vagina carved into his body to replace the penis. Within his fantasies, he was treated as a woman. This, in turn, activated the entire homosexual complex—including both identification with and desire for the father. Paradoxically, the malevolent traits he ascribed to female figures in his fantasies were ultimately projections of his father's attributes. Those who mistreated him personified the feared father figure, even though they appeared in female guise. Nevertheless, the patient derived sexual pleasure solely from the woman in the fantasy, suggesting that the father's role was that of the punitive agent—a projection of guilt related to his oedipal desire.

In this construction, the mother delivers sexual satisfaction through punishment, while the father enforces moral retribution. This dynamic opens a path toward homosexuality, although the gratification remained unconscious. The fantasy did not involve conscious desire for a male partner, yet the body part that gratifies the anus—namely, the penis—must, by definition, be male. Thus, the patient's homosexual orientation emerged not from romantic identification, but as a byproduct of unresolved anal eroticism.

The clinical paradox concludes as follows: the patient retained the anus as his primary erotogenic zone, mentally equating it with a vagina. Yet this imagined vagina must not, under any circumstance, encounter a penis. Were he to become aware of the identity of the "instrument" that satisfies this zone, he might consciously recognize his homosexuality and see himself as a passive pederast. To avoid this, his psyche constructed the fantasy of castration: by symbolically transforming into a woman, he evades the threat of recognizing the male source of pleasure. In this way, castration serves not only as punishment for oedipal desire, but also as a psychic maneuver to preserve disavowal: the man who must not be a man becomes a woman.

Upon reaching the discussion that followed Tausk's presentation, Eduard Hitschmann expressed that he found the paper highly interesting and, above all, distinguished by the richness of its clinical detail. However, he noted that its limitations lay more in the manner of presentation than in its conceptual framework—specifically, in its failure to delve into the deepest roots of the case. Regarding the patient's difficulties, Hitschmann concluded his remarks by suggesting that the patient's lack of success with sexual intercourse was likely due to the experiences not sufficiently corresponding to his internal fantasy life. Tausk acknowledged this point but clarified that the patient was not impotent *per se*; rather, what had been lacking was sexual sensibility. He traced the most fundamental causes of the pathology to two elements: anality and what he termed "constitution"—namely, a psychological predisposition anchored in the guilt complex. These two factors, taken together, formed the basis of the masochistic structure. As for sadism, Tausk deemed further elaboration unnecessary, summarizing simply that the patient had been an aggressive, sadistic child who had redirected his rage against himself.

At this point, Federn raised an objection, noting that Tausk had made no reference to his own earlier contribution on the same subject, presented at the scientific meeting on March 9, 1910. The presentation, titled "The infantile preconditions of masochism" (Nunberg & Federn, 1967, pp. 445–451), had previously outlined several foundational concepts. In response, Federn seized the opportunity to pose a series of pointed questions to Tausk, each deeply rooted in his own theoretical orientation. He inquired, first, into the nature of the patient's initial experience of sexual excitation—whether it had been centered on the anus, or whether it had arisen through penile masturbation or fantasy. He then asked under what circumstances the first seminal emission had occurred, and what illness had coincided with the onset of amnesia. Federn also wished to know how marked the patient's sensitivity to anal pain was, and whether anything of note could be discerned in the anatomical constitution of the genital organs.

Tausk replied by emphasizing that his clinical conclusions had not been constructed upon a predetermined theoretical framework but had instead emerged organically from the material presented by the case itself. He then addressed Federn's queries in turn: the patient's sexual fantasies had begun around the age of 6, and penile masturbation had developed concurrently with them; the illness that marked the onset of amnesia was pneumonia; although anal sensitivity had indeed been assessed, what struck Tausk most forcefully was the patient's pervasive bodily responsiveness, a kind of exaggerated hypersensitivity and ticklishness; and, finally, no anatomical abnormalities of the genital organs were observed.

Following these observations, Federn reminded the meeting of a point he had made in his earlier presentation: namely, that in individuals who later develop masochistic tendencies, penis-masturbation is often preceded by anal masturbation. In this regard, he noted that Tausk had indeed indicated that his patient engaged in later anal masturbation. However, Federn took issue with Tausk's assertion that the patient's passivity was not caused by the mother's sadistic behavior. This, Federn contended, stood in direct contradiction not only to the position he had outlined two years prior, but also to Alfred Adler's broader conceptualization. He maintained that Tausk should have addressed this theoretical discrepancy. According to Federn's clinical experience, it is often external factors—particularly dynamics of superiority and inferiority—that compel the child, typically from a highly sadistic family environment, to redirect their aggression into its opposite form. This, he emphasized, is not to suggest that such conditions are the sole basis for masochism; rather, they represent one necessary set of influences among others that must also be present for masochism to develop. Federn further remarked that Tausk did not draw a clear distinction between algolagnia and sadism, likely because in this particular case the two were intertwined. On this point, the editors of the *Minutes* observe in a footnote (Nunberg & Federn, 1974, p. 257) that although Federn refers to "sadism," it is evident from the context that he actually meant "masochism." The central question, as it emerged, was whether in the patient's fantasy it was the infliction of pain itself that constituted the source of pleasure, or rather the extreme and outrageous nature of the act. Tausk clearly favored the latter interpretation.

Another discussant, Sadger, stepped in to defend Tausk against Federn's criticisms. At the outset, he acknowledged several valuable points in Tausk's presentation. For instance, he noted that subordination in military service often acts as a precipitating factor in the onset of neurosis. He also underscored the frequent presence of a strict and controlling mother in the developmental history of masochists, illustrating this point with the case of the Austrian writer Leopold Ritter von Sacher-Masoch (1836–1895), whose literary explorations of desire, submission, and humiliation gave rise to the very term *masochism*. Furthermore, he found Tausk's reference to the "amnesia-boundary" being defined by a severe childhood illness to be particularly insightful. Sadger also concurred with the observation that patients often appear to be arrested at the pubertal stage in terms of their symptomatology—a phenomenon especially evident in cases of homosexuality (Nunberg & Federn, 1974, p. 257).

Nevertheless, Sadger expressed reservations about Tausk's contribution to resolving the deeper theoretical questions surrounding masochism. He suggested that masochism might be more effectively understood through the lens of erotogenic zones—specifically, the erotism of the skin, mucous membranes, and musculature. It is possible, he proposed, that the stimulation of skin erotism may occur without a corresponding breakthrough of pain sensations. Sadger concluded by situating the sadomasochistic complex within a broader literary and historical framework, identifying its most intense and intricate expression in the works of the Marquis de Sade, particularly *Justine* and *Juliette*. Allow me, before proceeding, to make a brief aside regarding de Sade and these works. Donatien Alphonse François de Sade (1740–1814), the French aristocrat and novelist, is renowned—indeed, notorious—for his uncompromising explorations of eroticism, violence, and excess. In *Justine, ou Les malheurs de la vertu* [Justine, or The misfortunes of virtue], first published in 1791, he portrays the ordeal of a virtuous young woman subjected to a relentless series of brutal misadventures, dramatizing the complex interplay between desire, cruelty, and moral transgression. Six years later, in 1797, an expanded edition appeared in the Netherlands under the title *La nouvelle*

Justine ou les malheurs de la vertu [The new Justine], which incorporated the story of her sister, *Juliette*, and further deepened the exploration of intertwined sadistic and masochistic dynamics (Sade, 1791/1995, 1797/1998).

Another discussant, Hanns Sachs (1881–1947), addressed the debate surrounding sadism and masochism by stating that he could not share the difficulties perceived by Federn and Tausk. In his view, sadism and masochism are, broadly speaking, one and the same phenomenon. He added that the patient described by Tausk bore a striking resemblance to Jean-Jacques Rousseau (1712–1778), the Franco-Swiss writer, philosopher, and naturalist—perhaps the most elusive and unclassifiable figure of the French Enlightenment—himself a neurotic haunted by unconscious anal-masochistic fantasies. What Sachs found particularly striking, from a cultural-historical standpoint, was that Rousseau—despite indulging in perverse fantasies—nonetheless set the template for the romantic ideal of love for an entire century, largely through the enduring influence of *Julie ou la nouvelle Héloïse* [Julie, or the new Héloïse] (Rousseau, 1761), a title that, however, appears in the *Minutes* simply as *La nouvelle Héloïse.* Moreover, Sachs emphasized that *Die Leiden des jungen Werthers* [The sorrows of young Werther] (Goethe, 1774) by Johann Wolfgang von Goethe (1749–1832), the towering German poet, playwright, and thinker, was the next seminal work to leave a comparable imprint on the cultural imagination. He noted that Goethe's novel, in turn, was profoundly shaped by Rousseau's *La nouvelle Héloïse* (Nunberg & Federn, 1974, p. 258).

In a subsequent intervention, Gaston Rosenstein (1882–1927)—who, after c. 1921, adopted the name Roffenstein—criticized Gustav Grüner (1885–1938) for having unjustly reproached Tausk with claims that did not in fact arise from the material. Freud then weighed in, remarking that it was inappropriate to invoke the contributions of Adler and Stekel in the way Grüner had done. Specifically, Freud objected to the tendency to credit Adler and Stekel as the "discoverers" of psychological facts simply because themes such as the masculine–feminine polarity or the feeling of guilt were mentioned—concepts that Freud saw as far more broadly grounded (Nunberg & Federn, 1974, p. 259).

In his final remarks, Tausk responded to these criticisms as well. He clarified that he had not spoken in terms of a desire to be either a man or a woman; psychologically, it had been sufficient for him to formulate the conclusions he presented. From Adler he acknowledged having only adopted the concept of inferiority, which he found to be particularly useful. As for Federn's point regarding anal erotism, Tausk confirmed his familiarity with the fact that anal expressions can manifest in sadistic ways—for instance, in fantasies of defecating in front of or upon women.

Approximately six months later, on October 18, 1911, Viktor Tausk delivered his next oral presentation, entitled "Problems to be addressed within and as a result of psychoanalysis." This lecture followed his earlier presentation of

May 10, 1911, discussed in detail above. He began by emphasizing that his remarks were not originally intended to conform to the prevailing conventions of academic discourse. A substantial part of his argument had initially been conceived as a polemic, but for various reasons, he was compelled to omit that portion. As a result, the task of demonstrating where and how psychoanalytic problems arise within the material had to be restructured. Tausk began with a pedagogical concern: how best to introduce psychoanalysis to students in a clear and accessible manner—starting entirely from outside its theoretical framework, without presupposing any of its principles. He posed the question of what kind of material could serve as an appropriate starting point. Although *The Psychopathology of Everyday Life* (Freud, 1901/1980a) might at first appear suitable, Tausk argued that this path already presupposes two fundamental psychoanalytic hypotheses: the existence of the unconscious, in Freud's sense, and the principle of inner continuity in associations.

From Tausk's perspective, however, precisely these assumptions render such material ill-suited for a genuine introduction grounded in "first principles." He likewise set aside other dimensions of psychic life—particularly pathological phenomena—considering them too intricate and conceptually demanding to serve as an effective starting point. Instead, Tausk selected the dream as a more viable starting point, one that could also serve his second aim: to demonstrate how, even in the simplest phenomena, psychological problems multiply and demand both scrutiny and categorization. From this basis, Tausk proposed that psychoanalysis calls not merely for revisions within existing psychological models, but for the construction of an entirely new psychology—one that both arises from and serves the aims of psychoanalysis. He warned that many problems psychoanalysis has addressed are now being "resolved" by academic psychology in ways that contradict analytic findings, and that still other problems are posed uniquely by psychoanalysis itself.

Tausk illustrated his thesis with a simple dream from a child, raising the question: What problems emerge from this psychic phenomenon when examined without psychoanalytic assumptions? He adopted only one working hypothesis: the principle of biological continuity between waking and dreaming states. From this, it follows that if mental life is a function of the individual, then the psychological unity of both states can be presumed. That dreams are psychic, not somatic, phenomena is supported by the presence of ideas and affects—expressions of specifically mental activity.

Hence, when comparing dream experiences with those of wakefulness, Tausk understood these as two distinct modalities of psychic functioning. The central task, then, is to uncover the mechanisms that differentiate these modalities. For such a comparison to be meaningful, a unifying category must first be identified—one that provides a conceptual bridge allowing us to move from the realm of waking life to that of dreaming. In this lecture, Tausk emphasized that his approach would proceed "from the side of consciousness." Since ideas, in his view, are abstractions derived from experience and must therefore originate in external reality—and given that, during sleep, no new sensory input from the external world is available—it follows that the content of dreams must necessarily be drawn from prior waking experience. External reality thus becomes the shared substrate of both dream and waking consciousness. This principle applies even to the most complex or seemingly incoherent dream content. Though such ideas may appear illogical or unrelated, they can be decomposed into elemental components, each traceable to real-world perceptual models. In the dream example presented by Tausk, he notes that the images appear to have emerged from waking consciousness without any qualitative transformation. As such, the question of a shared external reality becomes identical with the question of the dream's antecedents. These antecedents reveal themselves to be an unfulfilled wish from the previous day, with the dream's content corresponding directly to that wish and its attempted fulfillment through imagery. Although the details of the dream align with these antecedents, the overall dream scene does not mirror the totality of the prior experience. Instead, as Tausk observes, it appears as its opposite—evoking a parallel with a work of art. This leads to the simultaneous emergence of two types of problems related to thought (*Denkprobleme*): first, a *logical* problem, concerning the contrast between the dream's content and its real antecedents; and second, a *functional* problem, captured in the formula: "the dream is a wish-fulfillment." From this point, Tausk raises further questions: Do wishes exist in dreams? And what is a wish? The wish, he argues, bears a functional relationship to instinct, which he defines as a biological drive oriented toward self-preservation. Instinct seeks objects for gratification, while affect serves as a gauge, indicating whether a given object is deemed suitable for that purpose. Neither instinct nor affect tolerates delay in their relation to the object; they lack a *temporal* relationship, functioning only in spatial terms. This exclusion of temporality is particularly evident at a key moment in Tausk's dream example—when the affect associated with the dream image emerges. In the dream, the affect relates to its image as though the image were a currently present external object, ignoring the fact that the real object of desire belongs to the dreamer's past. At other times, the dream may treat future realities as if they were present. Thus, the dream is devoid of temporal awareness—it does not perceive the gratification as unreal. On the contrary, the psychological marker of instinctual satisfaction—*euphoria*—manifests in the dream just as it does in waking life. If euphoria is considered an indicator of a well-functioning organism, then the dream proves itself biologically effective in offering gratification to the instinct. But how, Tausk asks, can an instinct be gratified by an unreal object? Simply put: during sleep, real objects are unavailable. The instinct must turn inward, drawing instead on internal objects—that is, recollections. Through a unique psychic capacity, the mind imbues these memories with the semblance of current perceptual reality. Two psychic functions are at work in this transformation: first, the elimination of time; and second, the hallucinatory plasticization of the image. This second process—rendering internal objects with perceptual vividness—is itself a major psychological problem, one that Freud explored in his theory of the psyche's regression to perceptual modes. At this point, Tausk ends his presentation, noting that further questions cannot be explored solely through this single example, and that additional cases would be needed—though these fall outside the scope of his current discussion.

In the ensuing debate, Freud commented that psychoanalysis is, in many ways, the very last thing for which man is "naturally suited." Nevertheless, he emphasized that pedagogical efforts to present psychoanalysis are intellectually valuable and deserve our appreciation. Freud, also drawing on ideas from the influential German philosopher Theodor Lipps (1861–1914)—whom he frequently cited (Nunberg & Federn, 1974, p. 138) and who was a seminal figure in the study of aesthetics, empathy (*Einfühlung*), and the psychology of inner experience—explained the dream's capacity for hallucination by invoking Lipps's notion that the individual idea in a dream stands isolated, and is therefore no longer subject to the restraining influence of associative connections.

However, from Freud's perspective, this explanation invites serious objection: individual acts of thought are unmistakably present in dreams and cannot simply be dismissed as absent or negligible. Turning to the broader question of space and time within psychic life, Freud reminds us that the unconscious is, in essence, timeless. Yet this principle does not apply absolutely to the dream, which unfolds as a dynamic process between consciousness and the unconscious.

Conversely, space plays no role in the functioning of consciousness; it is for this reason that psychic phenomena often appear to us as having no spatial dimension. Time, on the other hand, is intrinsically bound to conscious mental activity. While the unconscious may lie outside the domain of time, Freud suggests that it nonetheless seems to retain spatial characteristics. Certain psychic processes, for instance, must be "reached" at a particular point if analytic intervention is to be effective. Thus, Freud portrays psychic life as operating in two distinct modalities: one in which time is absent but space persists, and another in which space is absent but time governs mental activity.

In a footnote to the published protocol, the editors of *Minutes* lamented that both Tausk's paper and the ensuing discussion were so heavily abridged that the immense richness of ideas originally presented was not adequately conveyed (Nunberg & Federn, 1974, p. 291). Furthermore, the editors noted that Rank frequently distorted Freud's remarks during the discussion—not deliberately, but nonetheless with substantive impact. In his closing remarks, Tausk insisted that he had been fundamentally misunderstood. His goal had not been to demonstrate how many conceptual challenges one must engage to approach psychoanalysis in a deductive, scientifically systematic manner. Rather, he had sought to illuminate the problem of time as it arises organically within psychoanalytic reflection on the dream. His reference to Schopenhauer was intended only to affirm that real perception entails both space and time. He did not mean to suggest that time is entirely absent in dreams, but rather that what is timeless is the affect's relation to the idea it accompanies. Tausk then addressed individual objections raised during the discussion, attempting to clarify misconceptions, refute criticisms, and remove what he saw as conceptual misplacements. Despite his considerable effort, confusion remained. Just two days later, on October 20, 1911, Freud wrote to Jung: "This past Wednesday I was once again able to observe just how much still needs to be accomplished here in terms of shared education" (as cited in Freud & Jung, 1974/1978, p. 516).

On November 8, Stekel and Reinhold, in their capacity as rapporteurs, presented a paper to the Vienna Psychoanalytic Society titled "On the supposed timelessness of the unconscious" (Nunberg & Federn, 1974, p. 299). Tausk was present at the meeting, though not among the designated speakers. Nevertheless, due to a clear editorial error, the *Minutes of the Vienna Psychoanalytic Society* (Vol. 3) erroneously list him alongside Reinhold as a presenter, omitting Stekel's name (Nunberg & Federn, 1974, p. ix).

Stekel began from the premise that the neurotic reveals himself as such through his relationship to reality. The neurotic tends to annul present reality and remain fixated on a historical one. For example, he may continue to love his aging mother as if unchanged by time. In this sense, the neurotic's infantile ideals are impervious to the effects of time; he remains in perpetual conflict with it, squandering time because, for him, it holds no value. The problem of time is also, Stekel noted, the child's tragic problem. The child, eager to "grow up," experiences time as painfully slow. The advent of the Oedipus complex then intensifies this experience: the child perceives with tragic poignancy the insurmountable temporal distance between himself and his mother. The feeling of inaccessibility—expressed in dreams and symptomatic acts—has its roots in this irreconcilable gap between child and parent, particularly the father, a gap that can never be bridged. Stekel even referenced a poem by a 6-year-old on the subject of vanishing time. Children, he observed, soon stage a form of competition with adults over this "head start" in life. Their mischievous satisfaction in having outlived their elders often surfaces openly at the latter's death. Yet this very attitude rebounds upon the child as a form of talion law, giving rise to the thought that he himself will die young—this being, in Stekel's view, a deep root of hypochondria.

Stekel went on to discuss the behavior of neurotic patients with respect to time in the context of psychoanalytic treatment: they arrive either too early or too late; they fear that the session will be too short to accommodate them. The significance of time also manifests in what he termed the patient's "unconscious calendar," which fixes certain past experiences and compels their re-experiencing on specific dates of which the patient remains consciously unaware. The neurotic's distorted perception of time is further evident in his impatience, his compulsive checking of the time, and his pervasive sense of having lost all temporal orientation. This tendency to "annul" the reality of time is rooted in the unconscious's refusal to acknowledge it.

When Reinhold took the floor, he sought to clarify the question raised by Freud regarding the timelessness and spatial nature of the unconscious, distinguishing it from related but extraneous issues. The difficulties stemming from Freud's assertion, he argued, lie squarely in the domain of epistemology—concerning the unconscious as an object of cognition. If the unconscious is conceived as psychic in nature, as psychoanalysis maintains, then purely conceptual reasoning dictates that one cannot deny that the unconscious knows time. To avoid contradicting psychoanalytic fundamentals, the discussion must exclude considerations of the temporality—or, conversely, the timelessness—of conscious and unconscious processes insofar as these concern the unconscious *as an object of cognition*.

Since Freud postulated the timelessness of the unconscious in contrast to the temporal orientation of consciousness, Reinhold proposed that one must first examine the complex relationship between consciousness and time. In respect to the organization of consciousness, he emphasized that consciousness is a purely historical construct—indeed, it is inconceivable without the dimension of time. However, it is essential to distinguish between an unconscious that is absolutely unconscious and one that is relatively unconscious, that is, unconscious only in relation to our conscious awareness. The unconscious may be regarded as a kind of historical personality that has become split off from the waking consciousness; as such, it too is bound to time, since its formation presupposes temporality.

Furthermore, the relationship between consciousness and time must be understood in terms of the limitations of consciousness itself: here, time functions as a conceptual boundary or limiting condition of conscious experience. In this sense, Freud's characterization of the unconscious as timeless and spatial is acceptable—provided that the term *spatial* is interpreted metaphorically, referring to the simultaneous coexistence of unconscious processes.

Finally, for the conscious psyche, the idea of time is a *conditio sine qua non*: it is the necessary precondition for all conscious experience. It would seem implausible, then, to assume that in the unconscious—where room exists for all manner of ideas and affects—time alone should be absent. The real question, Reinhold contended, is how the unconscious relates its contents to the concept of time: whether, and to what extent, it distinguishes past and future from present experience, and whether it can correctly orient itself with respect to temporal sequence.

Following Reinhold's exposition, Sabina Spielrein offered a noteworthy response, affirming her allegiance to a Jungian framework. She proposed that the unconscious operates along phylogenetic lines—a view that, in her estimation, explained the enduring impact of early childhood experiences on later psychological development. To illustrate this, she cited the persistence of phylogenetic elements in children's games, in sexual perversions such as inversion and bisexuality, in infantile sexual theories, and in the regression observed in cases of *dementia praecox* (Nunberg & Federn, 1974, p. 302).

Tausk and Federn, who spoke later during the same session, drew upon and developed several of Spielrein's observations in their own remarks. Tausk, in particular, emphasized that the discussion had, by that point, raised three distinct problems that bore no essential relation to one another, being connected only by the common term "time." He insisted that one must return to Reinhold's important assertions, which had approached the unconscious primarily from a cognitive standpoint—whereby it could be conceptualized only within the frameworks of space and time. The essential question, however, remains: does the unconscious "know" time? Do ideas arise within it in a temporal sequence, or do they not? Tausk referred to a previous remark in which the speaker suggested that affect relates to emerging ideas in a manner that reveals its indifference to temporal distance. In a psychic stratum composed solely of affects—according to Freud—temporal orientation cannot exist. The unconscious processes Spielrein had described as affective in nature thus take on considerable importance. For example, the unconscious lacks contrast because affect knows no criterion other than its own satisfaction. Its modes of expression do not belong to the affect *per se*. It is important to stress that we may, of course, later operate unconsciously on material that was consciously acquired.

In relation to this, Federn offered a clarification: in dreams, it is only the modes of expression that are substituted, not the underlying concepts. He also raised objections to Reinhold's methodological approach. From the observation of individual unconscious processes, Reinhold drew general conclusions about the nature of the unconscious—a move Federn questioned. He pointed out that mystics had long preceded psychoanalysis in their intuitions about unconscious timelessness. From their intimation of a timeless unconscious, they constructed a notion of eternity. Yet they were ultimately compelled to delimit this eternity by invoking a Last Judgment—because any attempt to apprehend the unconscious through consciousness is destined to fail.

Tausk then raised a critical question: Should the so-called timelessness of the unconscious be understood as a temporary deficiency, or as a fundamental absence of temporal orientation? In recalling a dream, for instance, we often struggle to determine what occurred first and what followed. Once the dream becomes conscious, it must be perceived within the framework of time. Yet due to the timeless character of the unconscious, it may in fact lack any inherent temporal sequence.

It is true, Tausk concluded, that in its deepest layers, the unconscious operates outside the dimension of time. It would be worthwhile, he noted, to investigate the developmental point at which the notion of time emerges in the child, for it is well known that children initially struggle to grasp temporal succession. In contrast to Spielrein's view, one must argue that the manifestations of the unconscious occur precisely *in the present*. At this juncture, we encounter the hallucinatory quality of the unconscious. The absence of temporal structuring within the unconscious is, ultimately, what makes sublimation possible.

Another participant, Rosenstein, challenged Tausk's thesis that affects are timeless. Affects, he argued, seek immediate gratification—thus introducing the factor of time. It is only our cognitive functions that are temporally oriented; other psychic processes are not intrinsically concerned with the concept of time. Yet the very notion of timelessness implies an engagement with the concept of time itself. Responding to Sachs, another discussant at the session, Rosenstein further objected that not every single wish or affect need be a derivative of the unconscious, nor should unconscious processes—as processes—be conceived as timeless. Drawing on the ideas of Wilhelm Jerusalem (1854–1923), a pedagogue, philosopher, and professor at the University of Vienna, Rosenstein noted that our concept of time is derived from the operations of consciousness—a perspective necessarily absent in the unconscious.

He maintained that Freud's statement referred to one specific characteristic of the unconscious: its unchangeability. Eternity itself is not synonymous with timelessness, as Federn emphasized; rather, it is the endless extension of time. Hence, one cannot properly speak of "timelessness" in reference to psychic processes; it is precisely because these processes do not operate under the governance of consciousness that they are mistakenly regarded as timeless. Conversely, the unconscious is far more susceptible to incorrect or distorted conceptions of time. As Spielrein pointed out, because the unconscious belongs to an earlier phylogenetic stratum of psychic life, it does not adhere rigidly to the structuring influence of time.

Rosenstein concluded that if Freud contrasted the timelessness of the unconscious with the temporal orientation of consciousness, his assumption rested upon a degree of separation between these two modes of psychic functioning that is, in reality, more fluid than sharply delineated.

At this point, it is worth offering a fuller portrait of Sabina Nikolayevna Spielrein (1885–1942), previously mentioned in these pages, whose prominent participation in this scientific exchange warrants closer attention. Spielrein—a Russian physician, psychoanalyst, and former patient (and intimate) of Jung—began her medical studies in Zürich in 1905, completing them six years later. In 1911, she defended her doctoral dissertation, "Über den psychologischen Inhalt eines Falles von Schizophrenie (dementia praecox)" [On the psychological content of a case of schizophrenia (dementia praecox)], which was published that same year in the *Jahrbuch* (Spielrein, 1911). Following a painful and widely publicized rupture with Jung—in which Freud acted as mediator—she married Pavel Nahumovich Sheftel on June 1, 1912 (Launer, 2014, p. 156), and the couple went on to have two daughters, Renata and Eva. Launer (2014, p. 157) records that Pavel was five years older than Sabina Spielrein, placing his birth in 1880, while another source gives his life span as 1881–1937 (JewAge.org, 2008–2025).

Between 1913 and 1919, Spielrein lived in various European cities, including Berlin, Munich, and Lausanne, before settling in Geneva. There, between 1921 and 1923, she served as analyst to Jean Piaget (1896–1980) over an eight-month period. His later interest in genetic epistemology and cognitive development, however, would follow a trajectory increasingly distinct from the Freudian psychoanalytic framework. Afterward, she returned to Russia, where her fate took a tragic turn. During the Nazi occupation, Spielrein and her daughters were executed—most sources date their deaths to 1941, though some cite 1942 (Balbuena, 2020). According to Appignanesi and Forrester (1992), she was shot on November 25, 1941, against the wall of a Rostov synagogue by German Wehrmacht soldiers under the command of Captain Fritz Neumann. Other accounts report that she perished on July 27, 1942, along with her daughters and many other Jews, who were herded through the streets to the city's outskirts and executed at the edge of the Zmeyevsky—or "Snake"—Ravine (Etkind, 1993/1997; Roudinesco & Plon, 1997). Her husband had died several years earlier.

Following this brief portrait of Spielrein, it is important to recall that she actively participated in the debates of the Vienna Psychoanalytic Society, where her presence often left a marked impression. Returning now to the records of the Society, we find that on November 15, 1911, Theodor Reik (1888–1969)—a lay analyst—presented a lecture entitled "On death and sexuality" (Nunberg & Federn, 1974, pp. 310–319). This presentation, building on themes previously explored in earlier Wednesday meetings, sparked a lively and wide-ranging debate among members, including Federn, Freud, Hitschmann, Rosenstein, Tausk, Sachs, Sadger, and Stekel.

During the ensuing discussion, Tausk sought to supplement Reik's theoretical exposition by deepening the psychological understanding of the act of love, understood more literally as the "enjoyment of love," conceived as an act of flight from the self into another. The mind that experiences existence as an unceasing struggle longs to escape the relentless awareness of that struggle—a release attainable only through extreme pleasure, through death, or, as Freud adds, through states of intoxication. From a psychological standpoint, Tausk posed a fundamental question: Is death to be understood as a symbol of sexuality, or does sexuality serve instead as a symbol of death? Both phenomena, he observed, fulfill a common function: they draw the individual away from the conscious awareness of the self—the persistent sense of "I am." Which of the two assumes symbolic primacy depends, in the final analysis, upon the unique structure of the individual psyche.

At this point, the discussion turned toward a theme of fundamental importance: the problem of anxiety. It may never be possible for the subject to be entirely consumed by the act of love, as a portion of the libido, understood here as affect, always remains unspent. It is this dissociated remainder that generates anxiety. Here, disunity arises: the unspent affect turns back upon the subject. If the affect has not exhausted itself along a single vector, orgasm becomes self-directed—hence, the link to death. In this framework, Christianity can be viewed as a cultural manifestation of anxiety to which an external object has been assigned. However, not all components of sexuality are equally capable of linking love and death; only those closely tied to the destruction of the subject—namely, sadism and masochism—fulfill this function. In this light, Reik suggested that "death for love" represents the masochistic equivalent of sexuality. Every life, he argued, is expiated through death; every anxiety, at its core, is a fear of death. At this point, the broader question of guilt arises. Anxiety, it would seem, is not produced solely by inhibited sexual libido; any obstruction of instinctual tendencies may give rise to it. Fear of death thus signals that the life instincts are being blocked—with the possible exception of the instinct for eating. Yet even the auxiliary instincts that eating shares with sexuality exhibit this same characteristic. In this sense, all anxiety may be understood as anxiety about death.

Spielrein, for her part, had already explored many of these questions in a work she had just completed and which would soon be published the following year under the title "Die Destruktion als Ursache des Werdens" [Destruction as the cause of coming into being] (Spielrein, 1912). There, she examined the fear of ego dissolution or of transformation into an alien personality; the problem of eternal life, illustrated through figures such as Glaukos Pontios, the Greek sea deity transformed from a fisherman into a prophetic merman, and the Flying Dutchman, which is experienced as equally terrifying as birth, with death itself representing another kind of birth. Spielrein also discussed the biological implications of these processes and explored death fantasies as forms of punishment for incestuous wishes. In her view, thoughts of death are intrinsic to the sexual instinct itself: it is simply a matter of whether the life elements or the death elements predominate—for example, in individuals who experience sexuality as a crime, such as in the case of incestuous fantasies.

Later in the discussion, Tausk added that this conflict ultimately arises between the demands of the species and those of the individual. The primary function of the instinct—serving the survival of the species—comes into direct conflict with its secondary function, the pursuit of individual pleasure. For this reason, individual gratification can never be fully complete. At the close of the meeting, Reik, then a doctoral candidate, was unanimously elected as a member of the Society.

Other sources indicate that Tausk praised the philosophical depth of Spielrein's arguments, noting that her approach was boldly deductive—unlike the prevailing inductive methods of psychoanalysis (Carotenuto & Trombetta, 1981). He also highlighted her crucial insight that sexuality is repressed in part because of its inherent destructive component. This observation would later be cited by Eissler (1983, p. 19) in his controversial claim that Freud believed Tausk suffered from orgasmic impotence, suggesting that Tausk's theories were based more on personal experience than on clinical observation. Marius Tausk—Viktor's eldest son—vigorously disputed this interpretation, insisting that his father would not have so markedly distorted reality (M. Tausk, 1983, pp. 304–305).

A week later, on November 22, 1911, another scientific meeting of the Vienna Psychoanalytic Society took place, this time devoted to the topic of masturbation. This was the first in a series of discussions on the subject, later published under the title *Die Onanie: Vierzehn Beiträge zu einer Diskussion der Wiener Psychoanalytischen Vereinigung* [Masturbation: Fourteen contributions to a discussion of the Vienna Psychoanalytic Society] (Die Onanie, 1912; Nunberg & Federn, 1974, p. 320).

During this session, Sadger began by stressing the enormous prevalence of masturbation, which he traced to three principal causes: first, the universality and intensity of sexual feelings in general; second, the particular suitability of masturbation as an ever-ready means of expressing any form of sexual pleasure; and third, its function as a source of comfort and sedation. In his view, the ultimate preconditions for masturbation lay in the inevitable excitations produced during infant care.

Stekel, however, presented a counterargument, citing as evidence the occurrence of masturbation among animals, which clearly cannot be traced to infant care. He noted that chance often plays a crucial role in the initiation of masturbation—people may discover accidentally that pleasure can be generated auto-erotically. Stekel also challenged Sadger's description of the so-called "masturbatory character," arguing that it is incorrect to speak of a fixed type. For instance, setting deadlines is not a typical symptom of masturbation; rather, such individuals often anticipate the death of someone close to them. As for therapy, Stekel stressed that one must take into account the fact that for many individuals—perverts and homosexuals in particular—masturbation may constitute the only possible form of sexual gratification.

At this point, Tausk intervened, affirming that Stekel had already identified the fundamental error in Sadger's presentation. For the problem, he argued, begins even prior to infant care; it originates in the instinctual life itself, which is oriented toward the pursuit of pleasure. The fact that this pleasure is sexual is determined by the organs of gratification; and the subsequent vicissitudes this pleasure undergoes are precisely what characterize masturbation. Certain pleasurable activities may outwardly resemble masturbatory acts. The "masturbatory character" is merely a special case; primary character traits develop from the instincts themselves, while secondary character traits arise from the vicissitudes of those instincts—in which masturbation, of course, plays a role. Tausk also pointed out that in the case of self-sacrificing women—those proverbial "aunts" who act as matchmakers—it is the procuring aspect of femininity that finds expression. To trace anal masturbation solely back to enemas, he argued, reflects a complete misunderstanding of the erotic nature of the anal zone.

Having outlined these points, Tausk's remarks opened the way for further reflections from other members of the Society. Of particular interest is the intervention by Federn, who criticized the overly broad use of the term masturbation. As a starting point, he proposed that its various meanings should be sharply distinguished: peripheral masturbation should be differentiated from psychic masturbation, and both from sexuality lacking a real object. Furthermore, a clear distinction should be drawn between instances where masturbation is a cause and those where it functions, to some extent, as a symptom.

Federn thus extended his critique by questioning the adequacy of the discussion concerning both the choice of profession and the supposed constitutional determinants of masturbation. In his view, masturbation is not, as Tausk had already emphasized, a symbolic action from the outset. At the same time, he acknowledged certain valid points—for instance, the links between deadline-setting, manual clumsiness, anxieties about virginity and fertility, and the passion for truth, connections that Rank had previously highlighted in relation to masturbation and lying.

At this juncture, Rank himself offered a clarification. In an earlier paper, he had sought to explain certain sharply defined character traits—such as deadline-setting and secretiveness—as products of the process of repression associated with masturbation. He emphasized, however, that his remarks had not been directed toward lying in general, nor toward pathological mendacity, but rather toward a very specific form of deception. The passion for truth, he argued, should be understood as a reaction formation against precisely this particular mode of dishonesty.

Once again, Tausk contributed to the discussion, this time addressing the term *pure*. He noted that in philosophy, as introduced by Kant, the word referred exclusively to the contemplation of function rather than its content. He further argued that philosophy precedes masturbation, arising at a stage when one is not yet aware of the sources of pleasure, prohibition, or inhibition. The very first exploratory impulse, he suggested, is already a philosophical one; subsequent specialization into particular topics is then shaped by individual endowment, and may even represent a reaction formation against a sense of inadequacy.

Tausk went on to propose that masturbation itself could be examined from three complementary perspectives: its causes, its aims, and its effects. Among the causes, he distinguished both external inducing factors and inner instinctual drives. As for its aims, one lies in the direct pursuit of pleasure, while another derives from the influence of specific inducing factors. Finally, the effects of masturbation, he maintained, can be both somatic and psychic.

He further suggested that the effects of masturbation vary depending on context and raised the broader question of its significance—within human society, across civilization, and in the field of medicine. To conclude the session, Freud remarked on the difficulty of determining whether masturbation ever occurs without accompanying fantasies. He clarified that this is not a question concerning infancy, but rather pertains to the period between roughly 3 and 5 years of age. The issue, he emphasized, must be formulated with precision: Can masturbation exist entirely without conscious fantasies? Freud concluded that this question could not be resolved without further investigation. In this regard, it is worth noting that the topic of masturbation would continue to provoke discussion in subsequent meetings of the Vienna Psychoanalytic Society, as already indicated in this account.

At the following scientific meeting, held on November 29, 1911, Spielrein presented her paper "On transformation" (Nunberg & Federn, 1974, p. 329), which she would later expand into her seminal essay "Die Destruktion als Ursache des Werdens" [Destruction as the cause of coming into being] (Spielrein, 1912), subsequently published in *Jahrbuch für Psychanalytische und Psychopathologische Forschungen, 4* (Freud & Jung, 1974/1978). In this work, Spielrein proposed that sexuality contains an intrinsic element of destruction, originating in the unconscious. When sexual desire is awakened, the ego—driven by the instinct for self-preservation—perceives this activation as a threat to its integrity and consequently represses it. In her view, sexuality is not expressed in service of the individual but is fundamentally in conflict with it—hence the necessity of repression. This theory offered a nuanced understanding of repression that should not be conflated, as Freud would later do in *Beyond the Pleasure Principle* (Freud, 1920/1979h), with a proto-concept of the death drive.

The primary point of contention in this session centered on the notion of ambivalence of desire, a concept introduced by Swiss psychiatrist Eugen Bleuler (1857–1939) and originally derived from Charles Darwin (1809–1882). According to this idea, every emotional state maintains a dynamic balance with its opposing force.

Despite the theoretical sophistication of Spielrein's paper, the presentation was ultimately judged unsuccessful: her audience struggled to grasp the depth of her argument, and the discussion became circular and unproductive. While Sachs contributed remarks on ambivalence, Tausk emphasized the metaphysical dimension of her theory—particularly the notion that sexual repression arises from a destructive impulse. According to the session records, Tausk expressed that he did not wish to base his critique of the paper on its specific content or material, but rather on the standpoint from which Spielrein approached her theme—a standpoint that, in his view, lay very close to the realm of metaphysics. He raised the question of whether life itself might originate by analogy with some older cosmic process—a question akin to that posed by Plato (428/427–348/347 BCE) concerning his inquiry into the world of ideas and the nature of God. From this metaphysical starting point, as Spielrein's paper had indeed illustrated, one could arrive deductively at the very questions psychoanalysis typically reaches inductively.

Nevertheless, Tausk recognized the significance of Spielrein's central insight: that resistance to sexuality may arise from its intrinsic destructive element. In his words, the entire mechanism of repression is fundamentally grounded in the fact that the death component gives rise to resistance toward sexuality. He drew an illuminating parallel with *Der Meister von Palmyra: Dramatische Dichtung in fünf Aufzügen* [The master of Palmyra: A five-act dramatic poem] (Wilbrandt, 1896). Allow me to briefly situate Adolf Wilbrandt (1837–1911) and his work. Trained as a philologist and philosopher, and active as a journalist and playwright (Randall, 1919, p. 58), he brought wide erudition to his literary production. *The master of Palmyra* presents a philosophical meditation on the tension between life and death, articulated through the poetic image of an immanent "over-soul" manifest in human existence. At its core, the play contrasts true immortality—understood as the ongoing transformation and expansion of the self—with the false promises of earthly eternity, embodied in Apelles, and the equally illusory Christian vision of heavenly bliss. In this way, Wilbrandt stages a dramatic exploration of mortality, transcendence, and the boundary between authentic and deceptive forms of existence.

Returning to the session itself, other members—including Federn, Rosenstein, Reinhold, and Stekel—built upon Spielrein's insights, using them as a springboard for wider reflections on the dynamics of the life and death drives and the origins of neurotic anxiety (Nunberg & Federn, 1974, pp. 332–333).

Later in the session, Friedjung criticized the increasingly abstract tone of the discussion, suggesting that it veiled a more profound, existential fear of death. In response, Tausk sought to clarify his position. He maintained that the ontogenetic problems addressed by psychoanalysis can equally be framed as general psychological problems. For the sake of comparison and conceptual clarity, he argued, it is necessary to draw upon broader psychological frameworks—where they prove valid—in order to provide the public with points of contact with psychoanalytic theory. Tausk cautioned that matriarchy, as invoked by Federn, remains a hypothetical construct. He maintained that such concepts take ontogenetic form through the individual's evolving relationship with the environment. At this point, Freud unexpectedly intervened in the discussion, redirecting it toward a critical examination of Jung's increasingly permissive use of mythological material in psychoanalytic theorizing (Nunberg & Federn, 1974, p. 335).

In the closing weeks of 1911, three additional sessions of the Vienna Psychoanalytic Society took place, with Tausk actively contributing to each. The first, on December 6, was devoted to a second discussion on "masturbation"; the second, held a week later on December 13, turned to the theme of the "feeling for nature"; and the third, on December 20, returned to the topic of "masturbation" for a third and final discussion that year. Although both the first and third sessions revolved around the same subject, each explored it from a different perspective and brought out distinct points of emphasis. What follows is a chronological account of the scientific meetings of late 1911, emphasizing their most significant and illuminating aspects.

At the scientific meeting held on December 6, 1911, as previously noted, the discussion returned to the topic of masturbation—marking the Society's second formal exploration of the subject. Hitschmann opened the session by affirming the universality of infantile and early childhood masturbation, as

Freud had previously demonstrated. This acknowledgment, he noted, had softened prevailing attitudes toward the practice and allowed for the insight that masturbation can, in some respects, be advantageous to the individual. However, he also warned of the potentially harmful consequences of excessive masturbation. Psychologically, the individual may be spoiled by the idealized fantasies it fosters, suffer from self-reproach over perceived weakness of will, and avoid the necessary struggle to attain a real love object—a struggle that serves as a model for later challenges in life. Such individuals often have difficulty enduring abstinence or coitus interruptus and may struggle with the transition to marital life.

Physically, excessive masturbation and the resulting increase in nocturnal emissions were linked to symptoms of sexual neurasthenia, as described by Freud. Hitschmann observed that many neurasthenic symptoms manifest analogously in women, who, he argued, engage in masturbation just as frequently and intensely as men. Among women, he emphasized sexual anesthesia as a major consequence, which Freud had traced to excessive clitoral stimulation at earlier developmental stages.

In the discussion following Hitschmann's paper, Federn broadly agreed with his arguments while underscoring the importance of differentiating prepubertal psychic sexuality from masturbation *per se*. He went on to question whether sexual anesthesia stemming from masturbation could, in fact, be distinguished from forms of anesthesia shaped by later psychic structures. He nevertheless maintained that every manifestation of anesthesia remains amenable to psychoanalytic treatment. Furthermore, he emphasized the need to differentiate the harm attributable to the act itself from that produced by the cultural construction of masturbation as sinful—in other words, to distinguish its immediate somatic and psychic consequences from those mediated through affective and moral responses.

Stekel, in contrast, was far more critical. He rejected what he perceived as Hitschmann's reactionary stance and argued that it is precisely among masturbators that one encounters expressions of genuinely heroic sexuality. Pleasure, he suggested, requires overcoming obstacles, and guilt often intervenes between the masturbatory act and its fulfillment. Stekel denied that masturbation causes neurasthenia and challenged the claim that it leads to sexual anesthesia in women. Rather, he argued, women masturbate because normal pathways to satisfaction—such as heterosexual intercourse—are unavailable to them, citing homosexuality as one possible example.

Freud contributed a methodological reflection, noting the complexity of the issue. He emphasized the importance of accommodating multiple perspectives and etiological explanations side by side, and of constructing a comprehensive schema in which the full range of relationships between cause and effect might find a place.

Tausk's contribution stood out for its effort to impose conceptual clarity on the discussion. Acknowledging the broad and intricate ramifications of the subject, he proposed a schematic overview—but not as a rigid taxonomy. Instead, his aim was to highlight how different aspects of the phenomenon could be addressed as interrelated components. He began by asserting the near-universal potential for masturbation to appear across time and place, and then examined its origins. The underlying cause, he proposed, lies in instinctual life—its demand for expression—while the precipitating factors may vary, whether external stimuli or internal reflexes. The function of masturbation, accordingly, is to obtain pleasure as a form of instinctual discharge.

Tausk distinguished between infantile and later masturbation, and between male and female patterns. He posed a subtle biological and psychological question: Is infantile masturbation merely a form of organ activity aimed at generating stimulation, or does it reflect a pleasure principle that transcends mere activity? This leads directly to the issue of when pleasure becomes autonomous from the function that produces it.

He also examined the diverse forms that masturbation may assume, ranging from genital and anal stimulation to the activation of other erogenous zones, from purely mental masturbation centered on fantasy to mutual practices, whether homosexual or heterosexual. Tausk devoted particular emphasis to the question of its effects, and especially to the possibility of harm. On the somatic level, he pointed to overstimulation of the peripheral nervous and endocrine systems, premature ejaculation, nocturnal emissions, and even impotence. Certain disturbances, he observed, may be transitional: physical manifestations such as lassitude, constipation, or anorexia can gradually acquire a psychic dimension. Yet for Tausk, the most consequential effects were psychogenic, arising less from the act itself than from the individual's subjective interpretation and moral evaluation of it.

These psychogenic effects included anxiety, particularly when the act serves only as a temporary expedient, and various links between masturbation and perversion. For instance, masturbation may manifest a specific perversion, act as a fixation of one, or even induce one. It may delay or prevent the choice of a real love object, especially when autoerotic gratification and fantasy reinforce an internalized, ideal object. This detachment from reality may hinder the integration of perverse components into normal love and result in the devaluation of women. In such cases, masturbation contributes to a cynical, objectless view of sexuality.

Tausk also reflected on how the masturbator's psychic economy affects character development. The tendency to revert to masturbation in moments of insecurity fosters emotional diffuseness, hypersensitivity, and a persistent incapacity for abstinence. The masturbator, spoiled by fantasy, often becomes overly sensitive to real imperfections in sexual partners, especially regarding the female body. This dynamic, coupled with repeated failure to overcome the habit, may lead to a pattern of resignation, self-doubt, and submissiveness—an internal drama that repeats across the masturbator's life history. Shyness, reserve, and despondency are also common traits. He noted, too, that the very struggle to relinquish the habit can itself provoke anxiety.

Finally, Tausk explored how masturbation may distort the relationship between the subject and the sexual object. For example, the genital masturbator, reducing the woman to her sexual organ, may quickly lose interest after gratification. This failure to synthesize the perverse component into a total love object leads to alienation and, ultimately, a form of cynicism. Here, Tausk implicitly returned to a theme he would develop further: the psychic economy of isolation and its consequences for love, attachment, and character.

Beyond these clinical considerations, Tausk extended his reflections to the broader psychological and sociocultural dimensions of masturbation, examining its significance for the genesis of neurosis, the dynamics of object choice, and the course of sexual development. One of the most significant effects, he argued, is the inhibition of sexual aggression, which arises from self-contempt and the internalized belief in the overpowering sexuality of others. The masturbator often feels that his impaired potency renders him despicable in the eyes of women—who he then imagines as sexually insatiable. This dual movement—both overestimating and underestimating women—reveals the contradictory emotional economy that masturbation fosters.

Tausk also observed that his excessive investment—hypercatexis—in the sexual sphere impairs not only his capacity for concentration but also his capacity for genuine satisfaction. Masturbation thus becomes a site of endless expectation: salvation is anticipated yet never arrives. The psyche, however, often seeks to compensate. Through rationalization and reaction formations, the individual may succeed, at least in part, in managing these impairments.

A further complication is the elevation of the love object into a saintly figure—a transformation based both on the maternal prototype and a compensatory idealization of the self. This splitting, or elevation, distorts love life by dulling the capacity for real sexual engagement and driving some individuals toward prostitution. In both men and women, masturbation can lead to emotional inconstancy: the real object repeatedly fails to measure up to the fantasy image. Love, thus, becomes unstable and idealization brittle.

Tausk also situated the problem and clinical implications of masturbation within the broader psychoanalytic issue of bisexuality. The male element cultivated through masturbation corresponds in men to a homosexual component; in women, the clitoris—a penis-equivalent—sustains a similar identification with a masculine, and therefore also homosexual, dimension. This latent bisexuality complicates the development of object choice and identity. Indeed, he suggested, one of the principal problems posed by masturbation lies in the fate of this bisexual disposition.

The connection between masturbation and neurosis, according to Tausk, is not merely causal but structural. Masturbation may act as a bridge to neurosis, but also bears a more specific influence on the *type* of neurosis that develops, depending on the erotogenic zone involved. In obsessional neurosis, the anal zone tends to be dominant; in hysteria, it is the genital zone that assumes primacy.

Drawing from 18 clinical cases, Tausk observed a recurring familial configuration: all involved sadistic fathers. In some instances, the father was overtly brutal and cruel; in others, he appeared as a remote figure of unassailable authority—omniscient and omnipotent. These different styles of paternal sadism, he proposed, played a formative role in the psychic fate of the masturbating sons. Remarkably, these sons had all maintained a belief in their father's asexuality well into late puberty. Around the age of 20, however, a marked emotional antagonism emerged—a reaction grounded in the father's failure to guide the son toward heterosexual love. The impairment of heterosexuality in these cases stemmed, in part, from the inability to sublimate perverse components and integrate them into the sexual act.

Under particular circumstances, masturbation does indeed become pathogenic—especially when the surrounding social milieu reacts negatively to the behavior in ways the subject cannot metabolize. Here, Tausk also pointed to constitutional factors, especially the intense cathexis of sexual need and of particular erotogenic zones, as mediators of this vulnerability.

Finally, he expanded the scope of his reflections to consider the broader cultural significance of masturbation. Certain forms of civilization, he argued, are intimately linked to masturbation—particularly when one acknowledges that many of those who suffer from its psychological consequences remain active participants in public life. For some individuals, masturbation constitutes the totality of their sexual existence. Prudery and sexual hypocrisy, in this view, can ultimately be traced back to the psychic structure shaped by masturbatory habits.

Tausk closed with a striking social observation: the general decline in sexual capacity, particularly among men, has contributed to shifts in gender relations. He even proposed that part of the emancipation of women can be seen as a reaction to this sexual deficit. A pervasive suspicion toward sexuality, he concluded, has resulted in a growing alienation between the sexes—a cultural symptom that, like many others, bears the hidden imprint of masturbation's psychological legacy.

Later in the same session, Tausk returned to the discussion from a slightly different angle. Following remarks by other discussants—Friedjung, Hitschmann, Sachs, and Dozent Zappert (1867–1941)—he commented on the psychoanalytic interpretation of thumb-sucking, emphasizing that the effects of early sexuality can only be properly understood through psychoanalysis. This, he noted, makes genuine dialogue with pediatricians particularly challenging, especially when they fail to incorporate psychoanalytic perspectives into their clinical framework.

Freud intervened at this point to lend his support to Tausk, stating that many of those present shared the view that the central problem in the choice of neurosis does, in fact, hinge upon the question of masturbation.

At the scientific session of December 13, the discussion turned to a markedly different theme: the "feeling for nature." Hanns Sachs, the speaker, began by applying the Freudian duality of the pleasure principle and the reality principle to man's relation with the natural world. From this framework, he proposed that human beings are drawn to nature through two interrelated aims: on one hand, the effort to master it—aligned with the reality principle—and on the other, the quest to derive pleasure from it, in keeping with the pleasure principle. This dialectic, Sachs argued, encapsulates what he termed the "feeling for nature," with natural science occupying an intermediary position that mediates and balances both principles.

Sachs located this feeling at the threshold of artistic reproduction of nature, identifying it as an aesthetic phenomenon that is more accessible to analysis than art proper, insofar as it is not yet shaped by highly individualized or stylistic factors. He illustrated its historical transformations through examples ranging from the Homeric epics—which embody the classical Greek rapport with nature—to modern expressions found in the works of Rousseau, Goethe, the Romantic poet and novelist Joseph von Eichendorff (1788–1857), and the Swiss Symbolist painter Arnold Böcklin (1827–1901). In contrasting these epochs, he traced an evolution in the psychic investment in nature itself.

Building on this historical analysis, Sachs contended that the feeling for nature functions as an expression of repressed instinctual life, with a particular emphasis on autoerotic impulses. This repressed material finds a displaced expression in the sexualization of the external world—a process that can occur both directly and via the detour of anxiety. The impressions of nature thus become charged with libido and are often personified, acquiring subjective qualities previously belonging to inner experience. Such personification, far from being a naïve projection, serves as a return of repressed autoerotism: the ego, which is prohibited as a direct source of pleasure, is externalized and then reinvested with libidinal energy through nature.

This mechanism, according to Sachs, is accompanied by a simplification of thought: the outer world is rendered analogous to the inner world, the primary object of observation. The resulting identification grants a form of forepleasure—*Vorlust*—a kind of psychic reward that prepares the way for deeper engagement. These libidinally colored natural impressions—now personified and invested—serve as vessels for unconscious fantasies, depending on the extent of repression and the symbolic pliability of the chosen natural object. In this sense, the natural world becomes a mirror of inner life, animated by the projections of the ego.

This entire psychic dynamic—the return to autoerotism, the splitting of the ego, the externalization of libido—bears striking resemblance to the processes found in mythology, and even more so, to certain psychoses such as paraphrenia—*dementia praecox*. For Sachs, the feeling for nature thus represents not only an aesthetic or cultural construct but also a regressive return to a phase that had once been developmentally necessary in the psychic life of humanity.

Turning to the modern experience of nature, Sachs observed that the contemporary sensibility no longer personifies natural phenomena as the ancients did. Rather, modernity emphasizes the subjective experience itself—the feeling for nature—while the object of that feeling becomes interchangeable and diffuse. In antiquity, projections onto nature were believed in; for modern individuals, by contrast, such belief is obstructed by the critical function of the ego and the dominance of the reality principle. What remains is a more abstract mode of affective projection, whereby we invest landscapes with "atmosphere"—a psychic coloration that lacks the fullness of gratification once achieved through mythic belief.

In this modern structure, repression has intensified to such a degree that the earlier mechanism of personification is largely foreclosed. What survives is a more subdued, symbolic interaction with nature—an aesthetic play rather than a psychic formation of social centrality. Where once the feeling for nature expressed collective fantasies and shared cosmologies, it now offers a private, often ironic commentary on our inner lives.

Briefly departing from psychoanalytic exposition, Sachs introduced a metaphysical speculation informed by Schopenhauer. He proposed that the sexual drive, with its latent ambivalence, could be understood as inherently incapable of full gratification. In this reading, the sexual instinct prevents the realization of the "will"—of which man is the objectification—thus reinforcing a condition of perpetual deferral that underlies both repression and sublimation.

Tausk, responding among the discussants, acknowledged the clarity and insight of Sachs's central argument but raised several concerns about its theoretical underpinnings. He questioned the use of "ambivalence" in relation to affect, noting that affect, by definition, implies a directed and decisive attitude toward an object. It was unclear to him what the term "ambivalence" denoted in this context. He also found that some of the presentation's foundational assumptions lacked psychological grounding—for instance, the notion that human development begins with the renunciation of pleasure, rather than with anticipatory self-protection against non-imminent threats. Furthermore, he challenged Sachs's developmental model, arguing that the conception of early human beings as primarily autoerotic stands in contradiction to Rank's portrayal of primitive man as generically sexual. The term "autoerotism," Tausk suggested, might apply to early humanity only insofar as we anachronistically impose on it a later concept, such as "infantile masturbation."

Sachs replied that many of these objections stemmed from semantic rather than substantive misunderstandings. In equating "autoerotism" with "general sexuality," he did not intend a narrow or clinical definition, but rather one that highlights the external world's function as an object rather than as a subject. He clarified that the role of self-protection had indeed been addressed within his developmental schema. Fundamentally, he saw his presentation as grounded in psychoanalytic principles, albeit ones still in need of refinement and elaboration.

Freud, in his concluding remarks, offered support and critique in equal measure. He endorsed the idea that animism arises with the onset of socialization, noting that this perspective could be corroborated from other angles. The neuroses, Freud observed, are of the same psychic nature as our highest cultural products; the difference lies in whether they are collectively shared or individually confined. Hysteria, he remarked, is individual art; religion, a collective obsessional neurosis; philosophy, a systematized paranoia. If the absence of the social degrades sublimated forms into neurosis, the force that replaces the social—namely sexuality—must be seen as the decisive agent.

Extending this framework to cultural history, Freud proposed that primitive man, in his narcissistic asociality, began to invest the world libidinally only upon entering social relations. In this transition, animism served as a bridge from inner life to collective representation. He expressed skepticism, however, regarding Sachs's hypothesis of an intrinsic ambivalence in sexual drives. While it is certainly true that the sexual instinct does not lead to complete satisfaction, Freud argued that this fact can be explained through its divergence from animal instinct—a divergence that constitutes the very condition for cultural development through sublimation. He cautioned especially against "handy" or speculative explanations of ambivalence, such as attributing it to the existence of two sexes. In closing, Freud reflected on the structural similarity between aesthetics and the practice of art—both being secondary psychic formations that became possible only after the decline of the animistic worldview. From this vantage point, no present phenomenon in the realm of aesthetics or symbolic life can be fully understood without reference to its deep historical and psychic antecedents.

Returning to the discussion, Tausk re-entered the debate to assert his claim to the idea that the sexual instinct is inherently incapable of providing full gratification—a point he noted had not been explicitly claimed as original by Freud himself. For Tausk, this incompleteness arises not from metaphysical speculation, but from a psychological structure in which each of the two fundamental instincts contains within it opposing and incompatible tendencies. These tendencies, though contradictory, are both subordinated to the overarching aim of species preservation. The feeling-instinct, oriented primarily toward the individual and only secondarily toward the species, is no less a source of inner conflict than the sexual instinct, which operates with the inverse priority: it serves primarily the continuation of the species and only secondarily the individual's needs.

Tausk also responded to Freud's earlier caution against the premature introduction of psychological presuppositions into theoretical work. While accepting the general validity of Freud's warning, he suggested that applying it too stringently would risk halting the very exploratory movement that psychoanalysis demands. Some degree of theoretical risk, he implied, is necessary if the field is to progress.

Having traversed these complex theoretical exchanges on the feeling for nature and the interplay between instinct, projection, and repression, I now turn to the final scientific meeting of the year—held on December 20, 1911. As previously mentioned, this session marked the third discussion on "masturbation," once again placing a core psychoanalytic theme under collective scrutiny. On this occasion, it was Rank who introduced the discussion with a concise overview of the psychoanalytic position regarding masturbation, focusing particularly on the genesis of the feeling of guilt. In contrast to prevailing views—which interpreted guilt as the product of external deterrents—Rank argued that guilt should instead be seen as a rationalization of the anxiety arising from unsatisfactory masturbatory activity, drawing an analogy to Freud's earlier formulation of anxiety neurosis.

In moving to the core of his presentation, Rank identified a set of psychic and characterological traits that may emerge in individuals who, while not overtly neurotic, have nevertheless been engaged in a prolonged inner struggle to repress masturbation. Among these, he noted the development of an exaggerated tendency toward secrecy—an expression, he proposed, of the private and forbidden nature of early sexual activity.

He further examined a peculiar variant of pathological mendacity: an obsessive compulsion to negate reality itself—a dynamic rendered with haunting clarity in the stubborn falsifications of the heroine of Grimm's *Marienkind* [Mary's child]. In the *Minutes* the tale is cited as *The child of Mary* (Nunberg & Federn, 1974, p. 360); in this book, however, I adopt the title *Mary's child,* which I consider closer both to the original spirit of the Grimm tale and to its stylistic resonance in English, reflecting the Grimm brothers' intent to preserve *Volksmärchen*—folk tales—rather than theological texts. Before engaging with Rank's interpretation of the tale, it is worth pausing to retrace its thematic contours, for only then can an alternative psychoanalytic reading fully emerge.

First published in the 1812 edition of *Kinder- und Hausmärchen* [Children's and household tales] by the Brothers Grimm—Jacob (1785–1863) and Wilhelm (1786–1859), the renowned German folklorists and linguists—*Mary's child* recounts the story of a young girl entrusted to the care of the Virgin Mary after her father can no longer provide for her (Grimm & Grimm, 1812). The Virgin grants her charge the keys to 13 rooms, forbidding her to open the last. The girl's curiosity leads her to disobey, and she is cast out of heaven, condemned to wander a life of hardship, marriage, and eventual struggle for redemption. While some later versions soften the explicitly Christian framework—replacing Mary and other sacred figures with fairies—the central themes of obedience, temptation, guilt, and restitution remain intact.

In his oral contribution to the discussion, Rank interpreted the girl's persistent denials as a reaction formation against repressed sexual truth. While this remains a fruitful reading, I propose broadening the interpretive frame beyond sexuality alone. Rather than viewing the refusals merely as a defense against forbidden desire, the tale can be read as an allegory of the tension between instinct and moral law, the psychic toll of repression and denial, and the possibility of reintegration through confession and symbolic mediation.

Mary here functions as a superego-like authority—simultaneously protective and punitive. The 13th door becomes a symbolic law, a primordial moral injunction within the child's psychic economy. The girl's transgression, driven by curiosity and the dawning impulse toward autonomy and knowledge, stages a universal conflict: the clash of instinctual drives with the prohibitions of internalized authority. Her repeated denials, and the punishments that follow—loss of speech, alienation, and condemnation—dramatize repression, projection, and moral anxiety in their starkest forms. Resolution comes only with confession and forgiveness, symbolizing the therapeutic process by which split-off elements of the self are acknowledged, reintegrated, and reconciled with the demands of internal authority. From this angle, the tale mirrors dynamics encountered clinically in neurosis, hysteria, and even psychosis, where guilt and denial must be worked through before psychic restoration can occur.

With this interpretive framework in mind, I return to the session's discussion, where Freud—responding to Rank's presentation—sought to restore methodological clarity. In formulating his critique, he drew explicitly on Johannes Jaroslaw Marcinowski's (1868–1935) essay "Zur Frage der infantilen Sexualität" [On the question of infantile sexuality] (Marcinowski, 1909)—by the Polish-born physician and early psychoanalyst renowned for his work on neuroses and sexuality—to contest Stekel's use of the term "*criminal*" in reference to objectionable instinctual drives in children.

Marcinowski had argued that such terminology was conceptually confused and clinically inappropriate; Freud echoed this point, stressing that "criminal" functions as a dense socio-legal construct rather than a psychological category and is therefore ill-suited to analytic explanation (Nunberg & Federn, 1974, p. 360). Furthermore, Freud observed that Stekel had failed to differentiate between infantile masturbation—occurring roughly between ages 3 and 5—and the adolescent form that emerges in puberty—a distinction essential to any coherent theory. In contrast to Stekel's attempts to determine whether specific symptoms stemmed from masturbation or from sexuality more generally, Rank—Freud noted approvingly—had rightly emphasized that masturbation *is* the form in which infantile sexuality manifests. Recent clinical observations continued to bear this out: for instance, Freud mentioned the case of a child whose compulsive pattern of "saving up" provided yet another link to masturbatory fantasy. Nevertheless, Freud encouraged deeper attention to the crucial question of whether the act of masturbation had been discovered independently or had remained secret, suggesting that this distinction bore significant psychological weight.

Federn spoke next, expressing broad support for Rank's position—particularly his view that masturbation should be understood primarily as a *symptom* rather than a root cause. Even so, Federn expressed two principal reservations. First, he argued that the presentation aimed to describe reactions in non-neurotic individuals, yet traits such as compulsive lying and stealing could not reasonably be considered normal. Second, he questioned the idea that pathological mendacity originates in excessive masturbation. If, as Rank suggested, obsessional "truthfulness" is linked to the successful overcoming of masturbation, then the variant of spiteful, compulsive lying described must be associated with a different dynamic—perhaps with the early need to conceal sexual activity. Federn cited two neurotic patients who, as children, had independently discovered sexuality and, believing themselves to be uniquely sexual, had grown up under the burden of persistent secrecy. For these individuals, lying was not yet moralized into guilt, but was instead a defensive adaptation to a world that did not yet accommodate their experience.

Tausk then shifted the discussion to Stekel's notion of the "criminal" instinct, criticizing its inconsistency and noting that Stekel himself had at times opted for the vaguer term "antisocial." In Tausk's view, masturbation in itself should not give rise to more than a limited range of symptoms; in many instances, sexuality seems merely to utilize masturbation as a transitional bridge toward the development of a social attitude. To illustrate this further, Tausk recounted the case of two brothers between the ages of 8 and 10. The elder showed no trace of guilt and remained unmoved by warnings about the dangers of masturbation, whereas the younger was consumed with guilt, denied his behavior, blushed, and became visibly anxious. Tausk explained this divergence by pointing to underlying psychodynamics: the younger boy harbored incestuous fantasies about his mother and a rejecting attitude toward his father, while no such conflicts were present in the elder. In this context, guilt is tied not to the act itself, but to the social prohibition—the relation to authority, to the law of the father. The difficulty in breaking off the habit without inflicting psychic trauma, Tausk concluded, suggested that masturbation might in fact fulfill a biologically useful function.

Elaborating his broader view, Tausk reiterated a principle he had often emphasized: that anxiety arises when libido is dammed-up or when the process of abreaction is insufficient. If a forbidden fantasy accompanies the masturbatory act, then the subject's concentration is disturbed, rendering the act itself ineffective in its aim. This inadequacy points to a deeper, perhaps intuitive, recognition by the child that some external object—most often a woman—is required for full discharge.

Rank, in response, reaffirmed his position. He had explicitly emphasized the role of object-seeking in the failure of gratification and the repression of masturbation. The objections raised had not disproved the spontaneous emergence of guilt; they had merely relocated the problem. Even if an external influence triggers the reaction, Rank insisted, it remains to be explained why such an influence carries such intense psychic weight for the individual. Tausk, returning to the terminological debate, remarked again on Stekel's shift from "criminal" to "antisocial." If sexuality is indeed framed as antisocial in this way, the child's sexuality itself becomes a form of rebellion against prohibition. Reik, taking exception to Tausk's formulation, challenged his characterization of the sexual instinct as inherently social. Tausk clarified his position: the sexual instinct, he argued, has both a social component and an egotistical one. In its solitary pursuit of pleasure, it is asocial and even antisocial—but when it seeks connection with another, it opens into the social sphere.

To close the session, Spielrein offered a reflective contribution. She found it difficult to determine whether autoerotism or object-directed heterosexuality constituted the primary condition. The child, she suggested, may be incapable of expressing overt aggression and may therefore identify with the powerful parental figures as a means of achieving gratification through assumed parental roles. The implications of this identification point toward both defense and development, the twin poles of psychoanalytic interest.

Three days into the new year of 1912, another scientific meeting was held—this time with Isidor Sadger as the presenter. His paper, titled "From Hebbel's childhood," was not fully transcribed in the *Minutes*, as its complete publication had already been planned. As the editors state in a footnote, Sadger subsequently published both an article and an essay on the same subject in 1913: the article, "Über das Unbewusste und die Träume bei Hebbel" [On the unconscious and the dreams of Hebbel] (Sadger, 1913a), and the essay, "Freudsche Mechanismen bei Hebbel" [Freudian mechanisms in Hebbel] (Sadger, 1913b). He further developed these ideas seven years later in his monograph *Friedrich Hebbel: Ein psychoanalytischer Versuch* [Friedrich Hebbel: A psychoanalytic study] (Sadger, 1920; Nunberg & Federn, 1975, p. 1).

Drawing on the autobiographical writings of the poet Friedrich Hebbel (1813–1863), Sadger examined his relationship with his parents, his early experiences of intense infatuation, and the connection—acknowledged by Hebbel himself—between his religious ideas and the father complex. These elements, Sadger argued, lent empirical support to psychoanalytic conceptions of the developing child's psyche and its internal conflicts. He also emphasized the close link between Hebbel's fertile imagination and his precociously awakened eroticism, as well as the states of infantile anxiety that accompanied them. Sadger concluded by noting that Hebbel could write such recollections only in a feverish state—a condition under which, not coincidentally, he often composed his most inspired poetic works.

In the ensuing discussion, Stekel voiced his reservations about analyzing well-known poetic works, warning against the repetition of the now-familiar mother complex in poets, since it is already known to be operative in all individuals. Contrary to what had been suggested, he maintained that religious dogmas do in fact leave a lasting impression on children, often producing a pathological effect in the emergence of neuroses—though such effects might only become evident many years later. The original emotional force of childhood beliefs, he argued, endures throughout life. For Stekel, the peculiar precondition for poetic creation lay in the fevered state itself, in which unconscious material could break through. With this in mind, Tausk found himself almost in agreement with Stekel's cautionary stance regarding the mother complex, and instead looked forward to a genuine psychology of artistic creation. Returning to Stekel's notion, he reiterated that the fever state may precipitate a breakthrough of the unconscious. This ties in with a recurring fantasy among young people: the desire to fall seriously ill as a way to stimulate creativity. Beneath this, Tausk suggested, lies a yearning to relive intense infantile affects—an effort to bring repressed childhood states to the surface.

Sachs, in contrast, underscored the value of such inquiries, emphasizing that, for now, they provide the only viable means to demonstrate that psychoanalysis can also serve as a psychology of the psychologically normal individual. The universal presence of a parental complex does not detract from the significance of a poet's willingness to speak about it—something the average person is less inclined to do. Moreover, this kind of childhood narrative is far from unique: one need only recall Rousseau, *Green Henry*, and other self-revealing autobiographical accounts (Nunberg & Federn, 1975, p. 3). To frame Sadger's remarks and the literary references he invoked, a brief note on Gottfried Keller and his novel *Der grüne Heinrich* [Green Henry] is in order. Keller (1819–1890), the Swiss poet and writer, first published the work in 1855 (Keller, 1855) and issued a substantially revised version in 1879 (Keller, 1880). This semi-autobiographical novel depicts a talented young man whose initial promise gradually dissolves into passivity and misfortune. Less a social critique than an intimate ethical meditation, it conveys Keller's conviction that character and fate—rather than circumstance alone—shape psychic failure. In this sense, *Green Henry* remains a profoundly personal document of inner conflict—one whose themes carry particular resonance for psychoanalytic reflection.

Hitschmann, for his part, criticized Sadger's uncritical reliance on childhood recollections presented long after the fact, questioning whether such memories could be regarded as objective or carry psychoanalytic value. He further argued that the work of greater and more self-aware poets might, in fact, be less amenable to analytic consideration. Hitschmann proposed for discussion the question of how the ideal love object is formed in very early childhood and whether the infantile object choice continues to function later on—alongside, and perhaps in tension with, the memory of the mother. Could it be that an erotic object exists even prior to the incestuous one? And if so, how is it that, at such an early stage, an erotic object choice is even possible alongside a love for adults that is grounded in caritas?

In connection with the overarching theme of "illness and creation" that framed this scientific meeting, it is worth concluding with a provocative observation from Stekel. He noted that the poet often enters a rapture of creation only after recovering from a serious illness—suggesting that those who confront death may seek to overcome mortality through artistic immortality. This underscores the importance of a deeper discussion around the psychology of illness. As the neurotic clearly shows, illness can bear profound psychological meaning. Hebbel, for example, presents a compelling psychological puzzle: his writing is perpetually shadowed by inhibition and rarely reaches the heights one might expect from his subtle and profound psychological insights. A week later, on January 10, 1912, Marcinowski presented a paper entitled "Drawings of dreams" at a new scientific meeting. Whereas the previous session had examined poetic creation and illness through the lens of Hebbel's life and work, this gathering shifted to the pictorial realm, considering drawings as expressive representations of dream activity. I now turn to the most significant aspects of that discussion.

The speaker presented a series of dreams, each accompanied by illustrations drawn by the dreamers themselves—individuals who, notably, were just as unaware of the symbolic meaning embedded in their drawings as they were of the latent content of the dreams. Through the analysis of this material, three core theses emerged. First, all landscapes and spatial settings in dreams are understood as symbolic reinterpretations of the human body. Second, these bodily representations ultimately point to fantasies concerning the mother's womb and, analogously, the father's "womb"—sites upon which the dreamer's erotic experiences are condensed. These fantasies are shaped not only by individual erotic history but also by the child–parent relationship. Third, religious ideas—far from being extraneous—play a central role in these unconscious formations, emerging as affective condensations rooted in early familial dynamics. Conflict, Marcinowski suggests, is the human condition: each inner struggle encapsulates both right and wrong, with God as the ultimate arbiter.

From this foundation, the presentation turned to the intimate relation between religion and erotism. This linkage is explored from two complementary perspectives. From a developmental standpoint, it is suggested that the fusion of the primal fear of natural forces with the reverence for sexuality gave rise to deities embodying both terror and love. The dying and resurrected God-Savior, for instance, symbolizes the phallus in its collapse and reanimation. On the individual level, this relationship reflects the emotional attitudes toward parental figures during childhood. A schematic differentiation is drawn between the sexes: women, owing to the configuration of their parental complexes, are seen as having a greater propensity toward piety, while men are more vulnerable to repression. The female libido is described as freer, less constrained by societal prohibitions—exemplified by the observation that female homosexuality is not criminalized.

After Federn and Hitschmann offered brief interventions, Tausk praised the paper's formal clarity and, in particular, the effective rendering of transitional phrasing and associative bridges—often a difficult task in dream interpretation. He also commended the interpretive courage required to draw out elements belonging to the dreamer's psychic life while remaining within the dream's own narrative frame. However, he expressed some skepticism regarding the unambiguous symbolic reading of landscapes.

Stekel, in turn, praised the paper's formal precision and noted that among the many poetic dreams he had collected, those set in specific landscapes carried the most intense emotional charge. He echoed Freud's long-standing assertion that all depictions of landscapes are maternal symbols. Stekel further expanded—or perhaps overstretched—some of the dream interpretations, suggesting, for instance, that large crowds in dreams often represent vast quantities of sperm. Like Marcinowski, he emphasized that sexual symbols are frequently inseparable from religious ones. In his view, the devout disposition of women is less a consequence of the parental complex than of their mode of apperception, which is based more on affect than intellect.

Freud then intervened briefly, affirming the symbolic reading of landscapes and buildings as representations of the human body—especially the genitals—as a principle that can scarcely be questioned any longer, though he acknowledged that the plasticity of psychic material always allows for exceptions. He challenged one point of Tausk's praise, stating that what the latter attributed to the interpreter was, in truth, the achievement of the dreamer and reflected a deeply individual process. Freud also noted that only educated individuals or physicians are likely to associate dream images of crowds with sperm. Regarding religious symbolism, he observed that the speaker had announced its significance but not yet provided adequate evidence for it.

At this point, Tausk asked Freud about the nature of libido limitations among so-called "primitive" peoples, receiving from Freud a hint about an ongoing work concerning the incest taboo—a clear allusion to *Totem and Taboo* (Freud, 1913/1980e) which first appeared in serialized form in *Imago, 1* and *2* before being published as a standalone book, as noted in a footnote by the editors of the *Minutes* (Nunberg & Federn, 1975, p. 11). Tausk then speculated that the repression of libido might be tied to the differentiation of the sexual instinct from the instinctual "heat" state observed in animals.

In his concluding remarks, Marcinowski explained that his inferences regarding religious symbolism arose less from isolated details than from the overall affective orientation of the dreamers. While he was already familiar with the earlier literature on religious imagery, he deliberately chose not to include it, given the particular focus of the presentation.

At the next scientific meeting, held on January 17, 1912, Isidor Sadger once again took the role of speaker. The discussion returned to Hebbel, this time under the title "From Hebbel's boyhood." What follows will highlight the most relevant aspects of this session, intended to deepen and enrich the lines of inquiry first opened in the earlier meeting of January 3, 1912.

Following up on his earlier presentation, the speaker draws on biographical material to discuss the poet's later attitudes toward his parents and siblings. These are marked above all by a growing strain in his relationship with his father and an increasingly close attachment to his mother. Hebbel confesses that it was due to his mother alone that he was able to resist the intense pressure exerted by his father, who had tried early on to force him into a career path entirely foreign to his nature.

Alongside the family complex, the religious complex plays a central role in the poet's psychic life. According to Hebbel, two roots underlie religious feeling: fear and the dawning awareness of a power greater than one's parents. The child accepts religious dogmas—which remain intellectually opaque to him—because, as Hebbel's notes make clear, such dogmas align with the unconscious in their enigmatic character. From these observations, Sadger inferred that the clinical picture pointed to an infantile obsessional neurosis—one defined by incessant rumination, doubt, and anguished reflections on nothingness. Throughout his life—as reflected in his dramatic characters—Hebbel seems to have experienced a deep need for self-justification. The speaker also posits that as early as his first or second year, Hebbel may have overheard parental intercourse.

In the discussion that follows, Stekel expresses greater satisfaction with the day's presentation. He mentions having compiled a collection of Hebbel's dreams, many of which revolve around the mother's womb. In this light, he interprets a childhood dream in which 4-year-old Hebbel is being rocked by his father and experiences anxiety. Stekel sees this as a dream expressing both repressed libido—manifested as anxiety—and a death wish directed at the father. The dream, he suggests, not only reflects the inversion of criminal thoughts into anxiety, but also contains the fantasy that the child in the womb participates in parental intercourse.

Federn raises critical concerns about both the style and substance of the presentation. While he finds the content largely accurate, he objects to the manner of its delivery. For example, the casual mention of the resurrection as a symbol of erection, although perhaps accurate for certain psychic and cultural strata, undermines the sincerity of the belief systems in which this view originated. Federn argues that religious belief in childhood does not necessarily stem from obsessional neurosis—just as identification with Christ can be achieved by any devout Catholic without indicating pathology.

Moreover, Federn notes that the real issue of sadism was not addressed: namely, whether it arises from early experiences of abuse or is rooted in a constitutional disposition. He suggests that early combinations of sexual sensations with corporal punishment—even when observed in others—frequently contribute to sadistic tendencies. In one case where such experiences were absent, anthropophagic tendencies, which Sadger also noted, were nevertheless present. Federn posits that individuals who stand out in any significant way often harbor the strongest and most archaic instinctual drives of humankind.

Freud, commenting on Sadger's presentation, expresses skepticism about the speaker's generalizations on religion. If religion were to serve as proof of the unconscious, Freud argues, animals—who function almost entirely through unconscious processes—would be more religious than humans. He notes that the fear of the nutcracker seems obviously related to the father figure and suggests that the common human fondness for caricature or the grotesque often signals an unconscious critical stance toward the paternal image. Regarding Hebbel's dream, Freud disagrees with Stekel's interpretation, stating that it presupposes the presence of womb symbolism that is not evident in the dream itself. Freud sees merit in Sadger's interpretation, though incomplete. While Sadger links the dream to overhearing parental intercourse, he does not derive that meaning directly from the dream. Freud points out that the dream's rhythm unmistakably mirrors sexual intercourse, and should be understood as a dream of overhearing—one marked by a particular complexity. The child responds ambivalently: on the one hand, wishing to take the father's place—reflecting oedipal dynamics—and on the other, desiring to take the mother's place—a passive, feminine position. Hebbel's dream, Freud argues, expresses a homosexual attitude toward the father—a wish to be used by him sexually.

Tausk offers a primarily aesthetic critique, objecting specifically to the phrase "wee Frederic," and noting that while the speaker is convincing when he discusses "primitive" or fundamental psychic truths, his accuracy diminishes elsewhere. Tausk challenges the idea that memory capacity alone marks the poet, insisting instead that it signifies intellectual capacity more generally. He affirms Freud's interpretation of caricature with a clinical example and adds that fantasies of burial often express love for the mother turned into hatred—many of these fantasies being, in essence, castration fantasies. The "torments of nothingness" are associated with three interconnected elements: first, the sensation of total emotional engulfment; second, the poet's reverence for an old book; and finally, his weeping for himself. This constellation of affects points not merely to anxiety but to a profound, drawn-out disappointment—a psychological state characterized by detachment from both past and future. During such periods, affect must operate to pull the individual away from himself, producing a peculiar form of *post coitum triste*, regardless of when it appears. The old book symbolizes an attachment to the past, while his tears reveal an acute awareness of his own misery. As the editors of the *Minutes* observe in a footnote, this portion of the discussion is difficult to follow—likely due to Rank's excessive condensation of material (Nunberg & Federn, 1975, p. 18).

In his concluding remarks, Sadger emphasizes that his discussion of religion was based strictly on Hebbel's own words. Responding to Federn, he denies attributing the features in question—such as identification with Christ—to obsessional neurosis. He also defends his style, noting that his published writings over the years have never provoked offense. As for the group's apparent resistance to his ideas on "hereditary taint"—an issue whose symptoms, he contends, are repeatedly confirmed—Sadger attributes their discomfort to unresolved personal complexes. The one-sidedness in his paper, he explains, results from omitting ideas presumed to be common knowledge within the group, though he had addressed these adequately in print.

If Hebbel was a recurring subject in two scientific meetings, so too was masturbation—a topic that received sustained attention within the Vienna

Psychoanalytic Society. In fact, beyond the session of January 24, 1912, four additional presentations were devoted to the subject: on February 7 and 28, and March 13 and 20, culminating in a final paper delivered by Freud himself on April 24, aptly titled "An epilogue to the discussion on masturbation."

Turning now to the session of January 24, it is worth highlighting the most significant contributions of that meeting, following the same analytical approach adopted thus far. Unlike earlier sessions, this meeting featured two speakers: Josef Karl Friedjung and Sándor Ferenczi. Friedjung opened the session by emphasizing the difficulties in collecting reliable material over the preceding year and a half. He noted that intelligent mothers and nurses, even when aware of such matters, tend to remain silent—thus complicating the acquisition of meaningful data. Nonetheless, some observations proved illuminating. For instance, the onset of repression—typically around the second year of life and often induced by toilet training—could be clearly identified in several cases.

In later childhood, Friedjung argued, particularly between the ages of 5 and 12, masturbation is often provoked by external factors such as balanitis. During this stage, orgasm is rare or manifests in disguised forms, and a resurgence of masturbatory activity frequently follows seduction by older individuals. Notably, extragenital masturbation—whether at the navel or through oral stimulation—is by no means uncommon, a phenomenon that Friedjung noted had already been observed by Lindner and Freud. Sámuel Lindner (1842–1911), a pediatrician from Budapest, is now regarded as a key precursor of the theory of orality (Kern, 1973; Sauerteig, 2012).

From a psychological standpoint, Friedjung stated that no Freud-style fantasies—at least not conscious ones—were observed during these later years of childhood. Nonetheless, a split in the personality became apparent, as boys who engaged in regular and diverse masturbatory activity still functioned flawlessly in their academic environments. Interestingly, boys who fantasized about women during masturbation often made a smoother transition to normative sexual intercourse. Friedjung posited that it is not the act of masturbation *per se*, but rather a particular psychic dynamic, that renders it pathological.

During the following discussion, Federn raised a compelling question: Is every act of masturbation accompanied by a sexual fantasy? He acknowledged that sexual discharges can occur through non-sexual processes, and while some may indulge in fantasies, others may not. Still, he conceded that children do harbor sexual fantasies, and whether these fantasies are consciously summoned or unconsciously sustained, the underlying psychic mechanism may be fundamentally similar.

Tausk emphasized the importance of empirical observation as a vital supplement to psychoanalytic interpretation. He distinguished between two types of fantasies—first, immanent fantasies, which are truly unconscious and cannot be visualized during the act; and second, parallel fantasies, which accompany the act in real time. The child often behaves "as if"—the masturbatory act corresponds to an implicit fantasy, and only later may that fantasy evolve into a conscious image, potentially becoming pathogenic.

Rosenstein, meanwhile, addressed the link between fantasy and autoerotism. If the fantasy involves another person, he argued, masturbation loses its strictly autoerotic character. Echoing Federn, Rosenstein viewed the unconscious not merely as a repository of the repressed, but also as containing innate psychic structures. However, he questioned the claim that infantile recollections could be retrieved through psychoanalysis.

Responding to Rosenstein, Freud clarified that the term "autoerotic" properly applies only to the first two years of life. Masturbation that occurs afterward, and is accompanied by fantasies of others, marks a transitional phase between autoerotism and object love. The precise role of fantasy in this evolution, Freud added, remains a key area of inquiry.

Ferenczi, the second speaker, approached the topic by excluding certain psychic disturbances associated with masturbation—such as those rooted in infantile castration fears or juvenile incest anxieties—arguing that these are secondary phenomena. Instead, he explored the direct link between masturbation and neurotic symptoms, presenting data on what he termed "one-day neurasthenia"—a condition that may later evolve into genuine sexual neurasthenia in the Freudian sense. Acknowledging the psychic component in *ejaculatio praecox*, Ferenczi also discussed the symbolism of tooth extraction in dreams, interpreting it as a manifestation of masturbation and, by extension, a symbol of castration as punishment.

As the discussion unfolded, Tausk aligned Ferenczi's perspective with his own, noting that the pathogenic impact of masturbation often stems from the absence of perversions in the foreplay, thus disrupting normative erotic development. However, the panel diverged in their evaluations: Stekel dismissed Ferenczi's remarks on one-day neurasthenia and morning libido as off-topic and inaccurate, while Steiner defended them as precise and relevant. Reitler added a counterpoint from his clinical experience, noting that the harmful effects of masturbation also manifest in cases of mutual masturbation between adults, where all the elements of intercourse are ostensibly present. This observation, he argued, undermines some of the assumptions made by both Ferenczi and Tausk.

In sum, this session—rich in empirical detail and theoretical nuance—reflected both productive divergences and shared foundations in the psychoanalytic understanding of masturbation, fantasy, and developmental conflict.

After discussing masturbatory activity for the fourth time, and in an exercise of intellectual versatility, the scientific meeting held on January 31, 1912, turned to a very different topic: "On the sensation of flying in dreams." The speaker was Paul Federn, who began by taking issue with Tausk's thesis that the psyche in sleep is identical to the psyche in the waking state. At most, he conceded, this could be true in a negative sense: the psyche of a person who is awake contains no ideational element that could not also appear in a dream. However, dreams contain elements completely alien to the healthy psyche in its waking state—elements encountered only in abnormal psychic phenomena.

Federn illustrated this with a case of neurosis, demonstrating the identity between the dream of flying and symptoms of dizziness. Based on his understanding of bodily sensations in dreams, he shed some light on the nature of conversion. He argued that flying dreams are based on a common sensation and, therefore, on a common fantasy, which in other cases is expressed through hysterical conversion. Conversion is a specific process through which such a fantasy gives rise to a somatic phenomenon—the reverse of a psychic phenomenon emerging from a bodily stimulus. Still, he noted, the feeling of dizziness is not identical with the sensation of flying. Consequently, the assertion that the waking and sleeping psyches are identical cannot be sustained.

To understand what was said earlier about dizziness, it must be noted that the transformation of some flying dreams into falling dreams can also be explained in terms of dizziness. Freud had already pointed out the connection between dizziness and childhood play—being tossed in the air and then dropped. The desire to act independently of adults is one of the roots of pride associated with flying in dreams, where it is invariably a personal skill. The sensation is received through the static organ, and the flying experience occurs via a regression to that organ. This does not, of course, exclude the possibility of psychic elements or input from other bodily organs.

Connecting the dream with sexuality, Federn stated that the end of an erection often leads to a sudden transformation of the flying dream into one of falling. The feeling of anxiety—traditionally attributed by organ theories to heavy breathing—is here interpreted instead as ungratified libido. Flying downward is understood as an inhibited sexual dream, corresponding to an erection that has misfired. He briefly mentioned additional sources of flying dreams: the desire to "outfly"; connections with flatulence and travel—as pointed out by Ernst Jones—and the symbolic use of flying dreams to represent death—according to Freud and Stekel. These various sources, he added, do not contradict one another but reflect the multifactorial nature of dreams. Nevertheless, erection seems to be the essential determinant.

In the discussion, Reinhold supported Tausk's position, arguing that what one experiences in dreams are images of flying rather than actual sensations. As a general principle, he noted that the real question is how vestibular sensations enter dreams at all—suggesting that, in neurotics, this may point to an underlying organic defect. He further remarked that the perceived direction of spinning cannot be changed at will and added, from personal experience, that he tends to have falling dreams when lying on his left side.

Tausk, identifying with the criticisms expressed by previous discussants, added that the image of flying may have been present in the dreamer's waking thoughts. In Freud's sense, he explained, regression stems ontogenetically from individual experiences. As for the idea that flying downward symbolizes inhibited erection, he remarked: an inhibited erection is no erection at all. He also referenced a dream that did not fit Federn's framework: one that begins with anxiety, and in which the dreamer feels too heavy.

Freud, for his part, considered the relationship between conversion and the flying dream to be the most interesting aspect of the paper. As a rule, only what is visually present in childhood memory can be represented regressively; formal and temporal regression usually coincide. Through the reworking of the erection stimulus into a flying sensation, the dream becomes sexualized; returning it to childhood serves the function of rendering it harmless.

He added that somatic compliance lies at the border between the psychic and the organic realms, and that the essential factor is the erotogenic disposition of the organ involved. In conversion, conditions of stimulation likely play a role. Even in physiological phenomena such as paralysis, Freud observed, the influence of psychic factors can be traced quite far. Yet, he concluded, the one-sidedness of somatic symptoms can never be derived from psychological factors alone.

Tausk, in this context, remarked that young children are taught to be proud of their bowel movements, and suggested that the relief experienced during defecation might also be one of the sources of flying dreams.

In his concluding comments, Federn rejected the accusation that he had blurred important conceptual boundaries. His intention, he clarified, was merely to show the connections with earlier authors and to demonstrate how, through the lens of psychoanalysis, familiar ideas take on new meaning and enable deeper understanding.

At the beginning of February—on February 7, 1912, as already mentioned—masturbation once again became the central focus of a scientific meeting. This marked the fifth discussion on the topic among members of the Vienna Psychoanalytic Society.

Before delving into the details of that session, however, a brief digression may be helpful here. In keeping with the chronological sequence of events, let me pause the account of the scientific meetings to turn briefly to a personal note penned by Sabina Spielrein just two days earlier, on February 5. As will become evident in what follows, life among the early analysts was not confined solely to theory or clinical practice; intellectual companionship often blurred into emotional intimacy. A particularly revealing moment is captured in Spielrein's own hand. In an autobiographical note dated February 5, 1912, she wrote:

> Recently, Dr. Tausk, after examining the lines on my palm, solemnly declared that at the age of 26 or 27, I would undergo a great event that would entirely transform my destiny. Jung married at 27. That age, therefore, shall be decisive for me. It is singular that Tausk could sense the decisive role he plays in my fate! If Jung's fate is linked with mine, then his double must be removed from the list of the living, for it is

doubtful that happiness strikes twice. Am I, perhaps, his tragic negative? To hell with it! Now, back to work.

(Spielrein, 1912, as cited in Carotenuto & Trombetta, 1981, p. 210)

In this brief yet evocative passage, Spielrein's voice resounds with her characteristic blend of irony, fervor, and psychological insight. Her words capture not only the personal weight she assigned to Tausk's palm reading, but also the symbolic triangulation in which she found herself—entwined with both Tausk and Jung in a nexus that transcended purely intellectual bonds.

Her striking remark that Jung's double must be "removed from the list of the living," immediately followed by a defiant "To hell with it! Now, back to work," dramatizes the intensity with which she experienced the psychic entanglements of love, rivalry, and destiny within the early psychoanalytic movement. Her reflection reveals a complex, ambivalent recognition of Tausk as a figure of transformation—someone who, like Jung, held a formative place in the architecture of her inner life. While her relationship with Jung had openly transgressed clinical boundaries and was saturated with emotional and erotic charge, her connection to Tausk appears more oscillatory—hovering between fascination and repudiation, articulated through the language of fate and mirrored identity.

Spielrein's self-description as perhaps Jung's "tragic negative" suggests not only a shadowed identification but also, perhaps, a premonitory awareness—conscious or not—of the destructive currents coursing through this matrix of transference. What surfaces here is a poignant glimpse into the crucible of early psychoanalysis, where theoretical invention, professional collaboration, and emotional life were inextricably intertwined. Spielrein, with striking lucidity, names the emotional stakes of a movement where love, ambition, and theory coexisted in volatile proximity. That said, I now return to the most significant aspects of the fifth discussion on masturbation. It featured two speakers: Rudolf Reitler and Wilhelm Stekel. Reitler's intention was to address only why masturbation can be harmful in certain cases. Before turning to his main topic, however, he criticized Stekel's assertion that neurasthenia is a psychogenic illness, emphasizing that not everything amenable to psychological influence must, for that reason, be considered psychogenic.

As Reitler argued, the wide variations in the psychological effects of masturbation among individuals can be explained, first, by differences in their psychosexual constitutions and, second, by the fact that a broad range of behaviors is subsumed under the term *masturbation*. In this regard, Reitler—drawing on the ideas of Leopold Löwenfeld (1847–1923), the German physician and pioneer of sexual pathology who, in his book *Über die sexuelle Konstitution und andere Sexual-Probleme* [On the sexual constitution and other sex problems] (Löwenfeld, 1911), criticized Freud's assertions—rejected the validity of inferring the nature of normal sexuality directly from observations of neurotic patients (as noted in Nunberg & Federn, 1975, p. 36).

Stekel, for his part, defines masturbation as any sexual activity carried out without the participation of another person, considering it, irrespective of the accompanying fantasies, to be essentially autoerotic—whereas so-called mutual masturbation does not, in his view, fall within that category. Thus, as Stekel observes, apart from certain harmful forms of masturbation that lead to disturbances in body chemistry—*Onania prolongata, interrupta, sine ejaculatione*—all other masturbatory activity is entirely harmless and free of ill effects; indeed, it may even exert a distinctly salutary influence. The typical image of the masturbator as mentally and physically deteriorated is a product only of outside influence, designed to frighten. Neurasthenia does not exist; behind it are hidden psychoneurotic symptoms. According to Freud, anxiety neurosis comes into existence only when masturbation is given up; usually, nocturnal emissions then appear, which in the majority of cases are masturbatory acts, on the principle of "pleasure without guilt." In this respect, the disproportion between masturbation and the sense of guilt is explained by the fact that masturbation is utilized as a reservoir for a great variety of feelings of guilt. The reason for this lies, on the one hand, in the teleological point of view, and, on the other, in the fact that in his feeling of guilt man creates an artificial resistance for the purpose of increasing pleasure. At this point, Stekel discerned a connection with religion. In his view, it was not Christianity that imposed guilt upon sexuality; rather, the pre-existing sense of guilt gave rise to Christianity itself. He added that, even when analysts succeed in persuading patients to abandon masturbation—a result not always achievable—the outcome is often more harmful than beneficial.

Contrary to Sachs, who has remained very doubtful of Stekel's presentation—especially on why it should be precisely masturbation, which is in and of itself quite harmless, that should become the reservoir for all feelings of guilt—Rosenstein finds Stekel's statement plausible. Tausk, in turn, takes up Rudolf Reitler's claim that toothache and intoxication—though organic in origin—can nonetheless be influenced by psychological factors. Pain, Reitler argued, becomes pain only when registered by consciousness; if consciousness functions merely as a sensory organ, one can then understand why, for example, a toothache might vanish through psychic influence. Tausk, however, admitted that he had never fully grasped the supposed primacy of the genital zone and, more generally, did not share Reitler's position (Nunberg & Federn, 1975, p. 38).

According to Stekel, masturbation indeed functions as a kind of reservoir, in which instinctual drive and inhibition can be seen struggling against one another. He goes so far as to claim: "It is the sense of guilt that has created Christianity," to which he adds that this guilt represents an artificial resistance deliberately "cut in" to counterbalance sexual life. Tausk, however, challenges Stekel's further contention that nocturnal emissions afford pleasure free of guilt; in his view, wet dreams are nothing more than intercourse dreams, apparently operating through reflex mechanisms.

As often happened in these scientific meetings, the intellectual exchange was rich and productive, with a range of arguments, sometimes converging and other times sharply divergent, offered by Freud, Rank, Federn, Spielrein, Hitschmann, Reinhold, Steiner, Bernhard Dattner (1887–1952), and Tatjana Rosenthal (1885–1921).

The next session, held on February 14, 1912, was presented by Karl Schrötter (1887–1913), a gifted young philosopher and one of the earliest to experiment with dreams. Tragically, he would take his own life not long afterward—the date of which remains uncertain. The *Minutes of the Vienna Psychoanalytic Society* place his death in 1913 (Nunberg & Federn, 1975, p. 43), whereas Eissler (1971, p. 283) situates it a year earlier, in 1912. His lecture, aptly titled "Experimental dreams," reflected his pioneering interest in the scientific exploration of dream activity.

At the suggestion of Hermann Swoboda, Schrötter devoted his presentation not to dream analysis but to dream synthesis, consciously abstaining from drawing theoretical conclusions. His experiments employed hypnosis, by which he induced a deep hypnotic sleep in his subjects—complete with total amnesia and loss of ordinary consciousness. Dreams occurred either during the hypnotic state itself or in the subsequent night's sleep. Importantly, the speaker reported no essential difference between the dreams produced under hypnosis and those emerging from ordinary sleep.

The experimental design comprised four main types, which Schrötter briefly outlined. First, in combinatory dream experiments, subjects were given several discrete ideas and instructed to dream accordingly. Second, in stimulus-based dreams, both mental and physical stimuli—real or suggested—were introduced. Third, in time-marked dreams, the subject was instructed to signal the start and end of the dream by raising and lowering the hand, thereby enabling a crude form of temporal measurement. Fourth, dreams involving thoughts, symbols, and censorship were induced by suggestions such as "dream the fulfillment of your strongest current desire," or other prompts referring to symbolic representation.

A common feature observed across most of these dreams was the frequent appearance of the hypnotist's figure within the dream content. In addition, Schrötter noted physiological indicators such as changes in respiration at the onset of dreaming, as well as dream-related bodily movements that corresponded with the narrative content, even when these had not been explicitly suggested during hypnosis. Drawing from a substantial archive of such dreams, and informed by his close knowledge of the life circumstances of his subjects—a 20-year-old woman and a 22-year-old man, both volunteering from scientific interest—the speaker traced the non-suggested elements of the dreams to residual impressions from the preceding day. No Freudian-style analysis was undertaken.

The discussion opened with Stekel expressing his appreciation for the speaker's contribution, even if it merely confirmed established findings—for instance, that the dreamer integrates external stimuli into the dream narrative irrespective of their nature. Stekel emphasized the value of having symbolism empirically confirmed by an impartial observer. Tausk, meanwhile, maintained that experimental and analytic approaches should be seen as mutually reinforcing. The persistence of dream censorship under hypnosis, he argued, offered a fresh perspective on the workings of hypnosis itself. Hitschmann, however, cautioned against underestimating the role of consciousness in hypnosis and underscored the experimental confirmation of symbolism as particularly important.

Federn also found the experiments highly promising, suggesting they opened a new path toward resolving long-standing problems in dream theory. From a slightly different angle, Sachs affirmed the symbolic dreams presented by Schrötter were of immense significance for psychoanalysis, even though they appeared somewhat closer to waking consciousness than typical dreams.

Herbert Silberer (1882–1923), a promising psychoanalyst renowned for his studies of symbolism and dream interpretation—and who, like Tausk, would tragically die by suicide at the age of 40 (Corliss, 2018)—took the floor to propose a distinction between two broad categories of dreams: those in which suggestion shaped the manifest content and those in which it acted upon the latent strata beneath.

Spielrein added a creative proposal: to suggest the same words to different individuals to observe how divergent responses manifest. One might also analyze a single dream and then present its latent wish to another subject, observing the varied symbolic renderings of the same unconscious material—some, for example, responding affirmatively to a homosexual suggestion, others defensively.

Reitler, in turn, was reminded of Jung's association experiments, seeing parallels in the stimulus-word technique employed. He underscored the value of such methods in verifying known symbolic meanings while also revealing new, previously unregistered symbolic expressions. Tausk contributed once more by suggesting that after dream production, one might ask the subject to reproduce under hypnosis the infantile fragments underlying the dream—though Freud, according to the records, remained skeptical about the feasibility of such an endeavor.

In his concluding remarks, Schrötter expressed gratitude for the stimulating suggestions he had received and stated his intention to incorporate them into future work. As for the question of "proving" symbolism, he tempered expectations, noting that his material dealing with symbolic disguise remained limited. He clarified his fundamental position on the nature of symbols: he could not accept that any content corresponding to a state of full consciousness be termed a symbol. For Schrötter, a symbol is a phenomenon whose entire meaning resides in the symbol itself, representing something that cannot be verbally articulated. Freud, as recorded, closed the exchange by characterizing this disagreement as essentially a semantic one—a dispute about words.

Turning now to the following scientific meeting, held on February 21, 1912, the focus would shift again. This time, the presentation was delivered by Theodor Reik, under the title "The parent complex as cultural ferment." In his presentation, Reik explored the relationship between the father complex and religious experience, emphasizing the extent to which infantile sexual curiosity shaped religious doubt, and how both this doubt and atheism could be rooted in the father complex. He then shifted his focus to the maternal influence in the development of the child, drawing on Freud's investigations into object choice—the "love type." From this vantage point, Reik endeavored to approach the psychological enigma of the Don Juan figure: a man who, on one hand, could not find enough women, yet, on the other, was perpetually unable to find the one woman he sought.

Reik suggested that the source of this restlessness lay in infantile complexes. Following Arthur Schnitzler's insights, he argued that doubt regarding women's fidelity had its origin in early childhood fantasies, which were also pivotal in the genesis of jealousy. Indeed, in Reik's formulation, the sexual jealousy felt toward the father constituted one of the deeper roots of ambition.

In contrast to Freud's typology, Reik proposed another masculine archetype: the man who desired only the pure, virginal woman—an idealized maternal figure—the "long-suffering one." This Gretchen-type, as he called it, was predicated on the unconscious presence of a third party who was absent. Its conditions were rooted in early childhood impressions, particularly in the child's wish to see his mother again as she had appeared to him before he became aware of her sexual being. In this construction, the mother was imagined as suffering, passive, and asexual.

When Stekel later intervened in the discussion, he characterized Reik's Gretchen-type as the bipolar complement to Freud's well-known type. Returning again to Reik's reflections, this idealization of the mother also underlay the figure of the "Madonna type," in whom the maternal and virginal attributes converged.

Addressing the parent–child relationship more broadly, Reik affirmed that not only must children undergo processes of detachment and renunciation, but parents too must eventually resign themselves. This parental stance often manifested in the model of education they envisioned for their children. According to Reik, it became increasingly evident that psychoanalytic insights needed to be integrated into the study of history. The generational conflict—between old and new, between tradition and innovation—the severing of ties with family and tribe, all testified to the role of the parent complex as one of the most potent cultural ferments in human civilization.

In the subsequent discussion, Tausk offered support for Reik's argument by providing clinical material. He presented the case of a 16-year-old boy with obsessional neurosis, showing how the influence of the parental complex could be decisive. If religion was not practiced within the home, the role of religious education in school became secondary; the religious teacher could not inspire devotion to a deity that the father figure failed to embody.

Federn, referencing the symbolism of the cross, remarked on the ambiguity surrounding its association with the notion of bearing a burden. Regarding the "Madonna type," he questioned the developmental period from which it originated, hypothesizing that it likely stemmed from the phase in which the child perceived the mother as asexual.

Turning to the core issue, Freud noted that the mother-type described was neither unique nor even the most common, but rather an especially vivid illustration. The ideal of the virginal woman, Freud suggested, might emerge as a reaction against the more familiar maternal figure. This led, he argued, to the broader question of the origin of all ideals: as both reaction formations and sublimations, they must arise from typical experiences and trace back to early childhood impressions. For Freud, the secret of love lay in the wish to be loved with the same intensity and devotion one had once received from one's mother in infancy.

Following interventions by Dattner, Hugo Heller (1870–1923), and Gustav Scheu (1875–1935), Tausk took the floor again to refer to an earlier work on the formation of the ideal. Through a specific case, he illustrated how the maternal image could displace the figure of God. He also raised the provocative question of whether Don Juanism might, at its core, reflect an unconscious perversion.

The subsequent scientific meeting, held on February 28, 1912—as previously noted—marked the sixth occasion on which the topic of masturbation was addressed. This time, the presentations were delivered by Maxim Steiner and Paul Federn. Opening the session, Steiner emphasized that masturbation should not be regarded as a symptom of illness—or, indeed, as a symptom of any kind—but simply as an activity: one among the various manifestations of sexual neurasthenia, which he insisted ought to be the true focus of the discussion. Given the difficulties that had arisen in earlier attempts to define a distinct masturbatory type and its corresponding character traits, Steiner proposed broadening the concept itself. His more inclusive framework encompassed not only solitary masturbation but also mutual acts, frustrated excitations, and nocturnal emissions.

On the question of whether masturbation is harmful, Steiner offered a clear answer: for the healthy individual, it is not, and in such cases, he argued, it constitutes a physiological necessity. The situation is markedly different, however, for the sexual neurasthenic. In these individuals, sexual function is altered by internal chemical conditions—linked to the endocrine system—such that the genital glands are prematurely stimulated. These subjects cannot tolerate sexual intercourse any more than they can tolerate masturbation. For Steiner, calling such a person a "masturbator" would be as misleading as labeling someone who cannot tolerate tobacco a "smoker." Masturbation, in his view, does not cause neurasthenia; rather, it aggravates and worsens a condition already present. In this way, Steiner lent support to Ferenczi's well-founded observation regarding the concept of "one-day neurasthenia." Stekel, however, would later, during the discussion, express his disagreement, explicitly rejecting both Steiner's position and the notion of one-day neurasthenia altogether.

Continuing this line of thought, Federn argued that, in the course of normal development, masturbation represents a natural consequence of the gradual maturation of sexuality and is generally innocuous. In fact, he suggested, it may even protect the child from seeking gratification in perverse zones. Whether or not masturbation is judged as harmful depends largely on its capacity to satisfy sexual excitation over a period of time, as well as on the extent to which the individual possesses alternative means of transforming or sublimating the sexual instinct. The longer the state of post-orgasmic relaxation endures, the more beneficial it becomes.

Federn's observations on guilt deserve particular attention. He pointed out that masturbation increases feelings of guilt because it involves acts of volition and concealment. Many individuals, however, do not become depressed due to guilt, but rather as a direct consequence of the masturbatory act itself. The harmful effects, he contended, reside to a great extent in the *aftermath* of the act. The psyche undergoes a significant shift: what seemed intensely desirable beforehand becomes, for a time, worthless. Having turned asexual, the psyche rejects the act that has just occurred and promises never to repeat it. This internal repudiation forms the precondition for guilt, which becomes more intense when instinctual suppression fails. One further consequence is that the aggressive energy of sexuality, left ungratified, turns inward against the subject.

Gaston Rosenstein, for his part, identified four distinct positions within the discussion. First, Freud's view: that excessive masturbation causes neurasthenia. Second, Stekel's rejection of the very concept of "actual neurosis." Third, Steiner's claim that neurasthenia results from an innate malfunction of the sexual glands. And fourth, Federn's belief that masturbation itself produces certain disturbances—though, in agreement with Stekel, he attributed these primarily to the role of guilt.

Tausk also took issue with some of Steiner's claims. The fact that psychological influence could be exerted in cases such as that of a neurasthenic patient suffering from neurotic constipation suggested, for Tausk, that something must have occurred within the psychic sphere as well—so that, ultimately, the issue remains psychological. He also emphasized the value of Federn's attempt to define the psychic structure of guilt.

Freud, in turn, offered Steiner a mixed response. On the one hand, he acknowledged that Steiner was correct in pointing out that the path to understanding actual neuroses must pass through an exploration of the somatic processes involved in sexuality. On the other hand, Freud outlined two major objections. First, that Steiner had prematurely settled the question of whether masturbation is harmful. And second, that he had failed to draw a sufficiently clear distinction between the sexual neurasthenic and the normal individual. Moreover, as Federn rightly noted, seduction can play a significant role in precipitating what is otherwise termed "congenital" neurasthenia.

Freud also described Federn's arguments as thoughtful but somewhat diffuse. Picking up on a line of thought reminiscent of Rank, Freud proposed that guilt develops in a way analogous to the development of anxiety: both originate from social feelings. The child first experiences guilt when sexuality is perceived as a social obligation. Where the sexual instinct does not orient toward any object, no guilt will appear. These social feelings, he maintained, are composed of egoistic and erotic components, and develop in part from sadistic tendencies. What is at stake here is a portion of the libido that, from an early age, has become bound to the ego instinct. The moment when this connection emerges depends upon the individual's constitutional makeup.

In response, Tausk expressed reservations about Freud's concept of "social conscience," arguing that it projected a later developmental stage into a primary position. If parents are understood as the child's first representatives of society, then the entire structure of guilt can be seen as rooted in the child's relation to the mother and father. Tausk warned against replacing a synthetic psychological factor with prematurely introduced analytical ones.

An extensive discussion ensued, during which Freud once more clarified his position. His intention in introducing the concept of social conscience, he explained, was simply to identify the constitutionally variable point at which sexual components become integrated with egoistic ones.

At the subsequent scientific meeting, held on March 6, 1912, the discussion took a markedly different direction. As the title of the presentation suggested, "A contribution to the psychoanalysis of traveling," the theme presented by Alfred Freiherr von Winterstein (1885–1958) departed significantly from the questions addressed in previous sessions.

In his lecture, Freiherr von Winterstein explored the various manifestations of the urge to travel, ranging from the spontaneous wish to travel to its pathological extreme: the fugue. Drawing upon psychoanalytic findings and numerous examples from the lives and works of poets, he attempted to trace this spontaneous drive back to psychosexual roots. Travel, he argued, is a form of motion that can offer a pleasurable discharge of motor energy. Furthermore, the sexualization of nature was seen to contribute to the pleasure associated with travel. In its pathological form, manifested as a compulsive drive to roam, this phenomenon was examined by the German psychiatrist Karl Heilbronner (1869–1914) in his 1903 article "Ueber Fugues und fugue-ähnliche Zustände" [On fugues and fugue-related states]. He observed that such travel was more often associated with hysteria than with epilepsy and frequently concealed deeper impulses, including criminal tendencies or even death wishes (Heilbronner, 1903). In every case, what was at stake was a temporary overpowering of consciousness by unconscious forces (Nunberg & Federn, 1975, p. 64).

Stekel, responding to the presentation, remarked that insufficient emphasis had been placed on the fact that travel frequently represents a compromise between erotic impulses and a desire to break free from the constraints of neurosis.

Sadger, in turn, regarded the urge to travel as a characteristic stigma of individuals heavily burdened by heredity. While his own clinical experiences largely supported Freiherr von Winterstein's claims, he also voiced several critical observations. He noted, for instance, that aversion to associations should not be confused with introjection; that an increased desire to travel in individuals with hereditary burdens did not necessarily stem from heightened libido; and that the longing for erotic experience, while certainly present in many cases, could not be posited as the universal basis for the travel impulse. In his view, the primary motive behind travel lay in the wish to flee from one's own tormenting ego. Rank, echoing this perspective, emphasized the theme of "liberation" as psychologically more decisive than erotic longing. He saw travel as an external enactment of an unsuccessful inner detachment. This mechanism, he argued, originated in the separation from parents and family that occurs during puberty—a model that would later structure adult behavior, especially visible in the neuroses of puberty and in the psychic life of poets as it relates to creative production.

Hitschmann, for his part, regretted the absence in the presentation of any discussion of the fear of travel or of kinesthetic sensation more generally—phenomena which he deemed intimately related to agoraphobia and to the very psychological motivations behind travel. He also pointed out that the symbolic meaning of travel in dreams deserved appropriate consideration. He questioned the contemporary custom of honeymoon trips, suggesting that if the urge to travel indeed stemmed from dissatisfaction, one might rather expect newlyweds to wish to remain in place.

Tausk contributed a clinical perspective by presenting two types of travelers observed in his analyses. In one case, the impulse to travel was a flight from a decisive confrontation with the father; in another, it stemmed from a desire to triumph over the oppressive conditions of the parental home. He identified the *Eternal Jew* as the archetype of the traveler—forever wandering in search of death. The incest complex and detachment from the family home, he suggested, were core elements of the urge to travel, exemplified in the case of a young man who, unconsciously, sought his sister in his journeys.

Spielrein observed, based on her clinical experience, that the impulse to travel can stem both from a passionate desire for detachment and from an intense longing to discover something new—a longing which, in her view, invariably conceals an incestuous motivation.

Finally, Freud himself shared a series of reflections on the topic. He proposed that the motif of traveling in search of a bride could be traced back to the earliest stages of human history, when, by custom, the father expelled his sons upon their coming of age. These sons would then travel to foreign lands, win a bride, and establish a new dominion. Fairy tales in which a foreign prince arrives to marry a local princess, Freud suggested, recapitulate these primordial conditions. On a more abstract level, Freud proposed that travel, as a symbolic act of separation, could plausibly be interpreted as a plastic representation of repression. He emphasized the psychological significance of space, pointing out that certain personality types—obsessional neurotics in particular—tend to experience a stronger relationship to spatial than to temporal dimensions. In some individuals, psychic complexes are displaced into external domains; emotional conflicts are projected onto physical localities, as is often the case with individuals who frequent spas or therapeutic retreats. In agoraphobia, Freud argued, such displacement takes the form of a symbolic transfer of sexual inhibition into spatial confinement. Through such mechanisms, the intensities of affect find tangible, external representation.

Leaving behind the discussion on the psychoanalysis of travel, let me guide the reader to the scientific meetings of March 13 and 20, 1912, which marked the seventh and eighth discussions on the topic of masturbation. The speakers at the first of these sessions were Hanns Sachs and Gaston Rosenstein.

Sachs sought to bring order and clarity to the still unresolved question of why masturbation, despite having a common cause, yields such varied effects. He proposed a twofold distinction: first, that masturbation could create a general predisposition to harm, and second, that under certain conditions, this latent predisposition might develop into tangible damage.

With regard to the general predisposing effects—those not yet fully explored—Sachs emphasized two significant aspects. First, masturbation lacks the instinctual condensation characteristic of certain higher psychic achievements. In sexual intercourse, multiple instincts—such as sadism, for example—may find simultaneous gratification. In contrast, masturbation, unable to channel all instincts through the sexual act, may force some drives to seek discharge elsewhere, as in the case of violent outbursts like prison revolts. Second, he addressed the difference between gratification in fantasy and gratification involving a real object. While normal sexual satisfaction involves the offering of an external object to the libido, masturbation entails a regressive movement: the object must be imagined, thus reverting to an earlier developmental stage.

Regarding the transition from predisposition to actual harm, Sachs argued that the specific etiology and manifestation of injury depend on the diversity of acts grouped under the term "masturbation." He proposed examining the phenomenon from three distinct perspectives. The first involved the nature of the act itself, taking into account the bodily area involved, the manner of stimulation, and both its quantity and intensity. The second concerned the psychic content of the masturbatory act, which varied depending on whether it was autoerotic or involved conscious or unconscious fantasy. Here, he noted that certain instinctual drives often cling to familiar forms of gratification that are comfortable, even when the rest of the psyche has moved forward. What may represent developmental progress at one age can become an impediment later, disrupting the proper distribution of libido—a disruption that, in Sachs's view, constituted masturbation's most serious consequence. Finally, the third point of view concerned the individual's relation to their social environment, as discussed previously by Otto Rank. A question was raised here about whether the seemingly lesser harmfulness of masturbation in girls might be due to the absence of a psychic correlate to the threat of castration.

Tausk, in discussing Sachs's ideas, praised the clarity and structure of the presentation, even if many of its insights had been expressed before, though not as succinctly. He found the term "condensation of instincts" at odds with the more familiar concepts of "confluence of instincts" and of the interplay among sexual components in the process of gratification. While overdetermination—such as an instinct attaching to a specific organ—was already understood, the notion of "condensation" might serve as a broader label for various forms of instinctual collaboration. Similarly, the idea that the masturbator must substitute in fantasy what a real object would otherwise offer was familiar, though typically understood in terms of incomplete abreaction. Prison revolts, Tausk insisted, could not be explained so generally; their roots lay in specific psychic conflicts. He also questioned Sachs's economic explanation of harm, arguing that, even in normative sexuality, the object must first be gained, and it is precisely the buildup of libido that allows for its eventual discharge. Nonetheless, he acknowledged the novelty and accuracy of linking masturbation with regression, and agreed that the failure to redistribute libido properly was central to its potentially harmful impact. Indeed, in every neurosis, the core disturbance lay in the persistence of infantile elements. Masturbation not only fixated infantility but also perversion—anchoring the psyche in an earlier developmental phase.

Steiner concurred with Tausk that, in terms of substance, the presentation added little that was new and had not resolved the crucial question: Why is masturbation harmful for some individuals but not for others? He speculated that its relative innocuity in women might be linked to their more developed capacity for fantasy, which would allow them to achieve psychic satisfaction with less energetic expenditure.

Federn intervened to correct what he saw as Tausk's misreading of the concept of "confluence of instincts." This, he clarified, did not imply, in Adler's sense, a collaboration between a sexual instinct and an ego instinct—such as sadism—since Adler believed that sadism itself arose from a confluence of instincts. While Federn acknowledged the validity of Sachs's comments on psychic economy, he cautioned against treating the dynamics of pleasure and unpleasure too lightly. Certain pleasurable experiences could, in fact, prove deeply harmful to the psychic economy. Moreover, what Sachs had described as a "permanent result" was not necessarily negative: in some cases, masturbation may even facilitate the repression of dangerous drives. The real issue was not whether repression occurred, but when the barrier to repression was breached.

By contrast, Freud endorsed Reinhold's argument that no true condensation of instincts occurred during sexual intercourse—only a condensation of outcomes. The term "confluence of instincts" was therefore to be preferred. Rosenstein, synthesizing the discussion, identified three principal issues: the characterological changes attributed to masturbation; the compulsive nature of the act; and the overarching question of its harmfulness.

Regarding the first, Rosenstein admitted to having no clinical experience. As for the second, he drew attention to a compulsive form of masturbation—sometimes occurring even alongside sexual intercourse—that he saw as rooted in an inability to integrate opposing psychological currents. This failure to synthesize, also evident in neurotic inhibition, applied to various conflicting polarities: love and hate—as seen in obsessional neurosis—sadism and masochism, ego instincts and sexual instincts, and, more broadly, instinct and repression. Freud, Rosenstein recalled, had shifted the focus from the notion of constitutional "disposition" to a dynamic understanding of the forces at play. Ambivalence, however, appeared particularly accentuated in the neurotic. When synthesis fails, the libido remains blocked, often necessitating a substitute discharge. Even when sexual intercourse occurs, it may be ineffective psychically, if it fails to engage the internal processes adequately.

On the third point, Rosenstein noted that the relationship between actual neurosis—with its toxic-autonomic origin—and psychoneurosis—of psychic etiology—had not yet been precisely formulated. Still, a kind of parallelism could be traced via the concept of inhibition or resistance—central not only to neurosis but also to the physiology of secretion. It is not anger itself that triggers this secretion, but the inhibition of affect. Rather than a motor response, what takes place is an innervation of the secretory system—thereby establishing a link between neurotic symptoms and processes akin to intoxication. Masturbation carried out under the influence of such inhibitions must produce effects quite distinct from that which occurs without them. The key question, then, concerns the nature and modifiability of these inhibitions: Are they more pathogenic when conscious or unconscious? Some may dissolve through simple explanation or psychoeducation, with the symptoms vanishing alongside them; others, like the more organic inhibitions described by Rank, prove more resistant. There are also biological inhibitions—teleologically driven—that represent yet another layer of psychic complexity.

Freud found Rosenstein's remarks on the connection between psychic and toxic phenomena particularly valuable, and agreed that the symptoms of actual neurosis could be viewed as symptoms of intoxication. Nevertheless, Tausk objected that what mattered most in neurosis was not merely that a striving be inhibited, but how such inhibition was utilized. He also rejected the idea that ambivalence alone could account for the totality of neurotic symptom formation; symptoms were not the result of two opposing forces from a single root, but rather of multiple and sometimes alternating influences. Reinhold supported Tausk in holding that neurosis was not caused solely by inhibition—though inhibition might, under certain conditions, be sublimated. Crucially, repression had to precede inhibition.

Having traced the main threads of this rich and multifaceted debate, my attention now shifts to the eighth discussion on masturbation, held on March 20, 1912, with Bernhard Dattner and Sabina Spielrein as the principal speakers.

Following the developmental trajectory outlined in *Three Essays on the Theory of Sexuality* (Freud, 1905a/1978a), Dattner delineated the changing role and effects of masturbation from early childhood through to sexual maturity. He emphasized the impact that both physical readiness and psychic development exert on the nature and consequences of masturbatory behavior. In early childhood, such activity is seen as serving biological interests and is considered largely harmless—unless practiced excessively or inhibited by traumatic prohibitions. It is typically during the latency period, when the first psychic barriers to sexuality are erected, that signs of psychological and physical harm begin to appear.

However, the most significant consequences, Dattner argued, manifest during puberty. At this stage, stimulation of any erotogenic zone may prove harmful, though genital masturbation is regarded as more deleterious than extragenital forms due to the associated loss of semen. *Mental masturbation*, in turn, is deemed even more detrimental than manual stimulation, as it engages the psyche with greater intensity. An instinctive awareness of the act's incompatibility with species propagation, combined with its frequency, may further exacerbate these adverse effects. Dattner also suggested a connection between habitual masturbation, diminished willpower, and disturbances in internal secretion. Overall, he viewed masturbation as an unfortunate yet inevitable accompaniment of puberty—its harmfulness lying less in the act itself than in a constitutionally inferior *Anlage.*

Federn, while largely agreeing, challenged several of Dattner's assertions. He noted that the idea of genital development continuing during the latency period was a misleading formulation; more accurately, when genital maturation intensifies, latency itself is interrupted. He further rejected the notion that semen loss or forceful ejaculation constitutes harm in itself. Given the variety of factors proposed throughout the discussion, he argued, it is insufficient to single out one type of masturbation as more damaging than another.

Tausk also took issue with certain premises. Sexual activity, he argued, does not serve biological interests *only* in early childhood—it does so throughout life. Moreover, he contended that disgust, shame, and morality cannot be uniformly subsumed under the category of "sublimation," since each stems from distinct origins. Tausk also questioned the common assumption that masturbation ceases entirely during the latency period, noting that this does not align with clinical observations.

Responding to this, Sachs clarified Freud's position: during latency, sexual activity does not halt but rather becomes stationary—it does not evolve further. He highlighted a temporal distinction in the psychic economy of sexual release: in coitus, psychic investment intensifies before the act, whereas in masturbation, fantasy must be sustained at the very peak of sexual tension.

Hitschmann added that the term "latency" is too often taken literally; it signifies, rather, the temporary disappearance of *manifest* masturbatory activity. Tausk pressed further for clarification of the term "psychic masturbation," defining it as fantasy-driven stimulation leading to ejaculation—a practice he believed particularly harmful to the psyche's safety valve, and one that may contribute to *ejaculatio praecox*.

In another of his interventions, Tausk suggested that the heightened amnesia surrounding masturbation during this period stems from the emergence of shame, which in turn reflects an internal recognition that there is something to be ashamed of—thus affirming the persistence of the activity, even if unconsciously repressed.

Spielrein noted the continued ambiguity in how masturbation is defined, pointing to the multiplicity of clinical observations. In girls, she argued, it often takes less visible forms, such as the pleasurable retention of natural bodily needs. Feelings of guilt tend to be intertwined with religious ideas. Spielrein also proposed an analogy: just as men harbor castration fantasies, women may project analogous fantasies onto men. She cited patients who feared that their hands would fall off or who harbored fantasies of strangulation. One superstition she mentioned involved the sensation of "having one's mind sewn shut." Additionally, Spielrein reported that in some cases the desire for masturbation was triggered by kleptomania.

Hitschmann, from a different angle, referred to masturbation following anxiety states or triggered by reading romantic novels. He proposed a typology of music: one kind serving a cathartic function, and another acting as a source of excitation—noting that playing the piano in dreams frequently symbolizes masturbation. He called for a closer examination of the connection between musicians and neurotics.

On this point, Tausk added that music represents a level of human expression that precedes conceptual thought—where abreaction occurs purely through the release of affect. Music that stimulates associations operates differently. He also referred to a feminine counterpart to the male castration fantasy—namely, fantasies of biting off the male organ—an image he associated with themes of threatened virility and reproductive anxiety in Émile Zola's novel *Fécondité* [Fecundity] (Zola, 1899). In that work, Émile Zola (1840–1902)—the eminent French novelist, essayist, and leading figure of literary naturalism, whose influence extended from fiction to the modern stage—dramatizes the conflict between fecundity and sterility, exalting procreation as a regenerative force while portraying voluntary infertility as a manifestation of egoism, degeneration, and psychic misery (Zola, 1899). For Tausk, such imagery underscores how passive castration fantasies may assume a distinct psychic function, linked not only to loss and mutilation but also, symbolically, to the act of birth. He further suggested that the castration fantasy may be phylogenetically rooted and, in certain neurotic configurations, bound to the dialectic between destruction and renewal. Tausk cited a case where kleptomania followed forbidden sexual acts, and Rank expanded on this, proposing that while the forbidden content of the kleptomaniac act may vary, its mechanism often mimics that of masturbation.

Freud ultimately advised caution in efforts to construct a female analog to the male castration fantasy. For him, the woman has no need to produce such a fantasy—she enters the world already *castrated*, as a woman. At most, she later endorses this reality through the fantasy that her penis has been cut off.

One week later, on March 27, 1912, Viktor Tausk—one of the Society's most active participants—took the floor as speaker. The topic of his presentation was titled "Sexuality and the ego." What follows is a brief overview of the most salient points addressed during the session. In his presentation, Tausk examined the two principal classes of instincts then recognized: ego instinct and sexual instinct. He focused in particular on sadism, which he interpreted as a fusion of both. In his analysis, sadism emerged as a distinctly masculine expression of aggression and control. This perspective resonated with Spielrein's prior suggestion that masochism, by contrast, bore a feminine psychological structure.

In the discussion that followed Tausk's presentation, Spielrein took the floor to argue that the repression of sexuality stems from the fundamentally bipolar nature of the sexual drive—it harbors within itself the potential for a total dissolution of the ego. Accordingly, she contended that when Tausk claimed the ego disintegrates during the sexual act, he was, in effect, restating her own theoretical position.

Subsequently, in the same session—following Tausk's presentation and Spielrein's remarks—significant contributions to the discussion were made by both Stekel and Freud. Stekel took the floor first, challenging the foundational dichotomy proposed by Tausk between ego instincts and sexual instincts. He regarded this contrast as artificial, asserting instead that the sexual instinct was in fact the most powerful among the ego instincts. According to Stekel, all instinctual life is by nature unconscious, and it is erroneous to define ego instincts merely as those drives that have been accepted by consciousness. A powerful affect, rather than dissolving the ego, awakens it—albeit the unconscious ego, the same psychic instance that emerges during orgasm. He also contested any proposed link between sadism and constipation, arguing that analytical experience reveals entirely different associative pathways. Similarly, he reaffirmed, as Rosenstein had previously noted, that contraceptive practices do not, in and of themselves, result in anxiety neuroses.

Freud followed, contributing a more nuanced metapsychological and epistemological perspective. He acknowledged the philosophical naïveté inherent in early psychoanalytic conceptualization, noting that its categories arose not from philosophical deduction but from clinical observation—specifically, from the empirical finding that neurotic symptoms often stem from repressed sexual components. The remainder of instinctual life was subsequently grouped under the provisional rubric of "ego instincts." Freud reminded the audience that psychoanalysis, in its early theoretical stages, must necessarily work with vague and provisional concepts, only later delineating their boundaries with greater precision. He aligned himself with Reinhold's suggestion that "instinct" should be treated as a hypothetical construct, situated at the interface of the psychic and the somatic. In this light, Stekel's position—assigning the sexual instinct to the domain of the ego—did not fundamentally contradict Tausk's, since the latter had already emphasized the intrinsic proximity of the two instinctual groups. Freud proposed a historical analogy: all intrapsychic conflict was once intersubjective. What appears today as a psychic defense mounted by the ego against sexuality was, in earlier times, an external conflict that had been internalized over the course of development.

Regarding sadism, Freud cautioned that no definitive conclusions could yet be drawn about its role as a point of convergence between ego and sexual instincts. He did, however, identify a more essential interface between the two: the stage of narcissism, wherein the totality of the libido is cathected onto the ego. It is from this moment onward that the differentiation between instinctual domains becomes more clearly discernible. Freud agreed with Spielrein's earlier formulation that the problem of sadomasochism is structurally identical with that of the instinct of destruction. Nevertheless, he reiterated his skepticism about linking sadism to physiological symptoms such as constipation, noting that such associations remain too tenuous and premature to support any definitive theoretical judgment.

Following Freud's intervention, a dialectical exchange unfolded between him and Stekel concerning the theoretical foundations of repression. Stekel voiced certain reservations about Freud's ingenious hypothesis and advanced a more straightforward explanatory principle: that repression operates in the service of enhancing pleasure. As Stekel contended, once the external world ceases to impose sufficient constraints, repression arises internally to preserve the requisite tension—thereby allowing pleasure to intensify. In his view, the internal barriers constructed through repression are themselves products of the pleasure principle. Freud countered this by asserting that such a mechanism—resistance introduced for the sake of increasing pleasure—occurs only in the domain of the sexual instinct. Stekel, however, challenged this limitation, suggesting that the same process can be observed in behaviors such as abstinence in drinkers or moderation in eaters, indicating its broader applicability beyond sexuality.

Federn then offered a critique of Tausk's presentation. He found no overt philosophical speculation in it but took issue with Tausk's claim that the sexual instinct primarily serves the preservation of the species. For Federn, the only human instinct that directly fulfills that function is the maternal instinct. He argued that comparisons between ego and sexual instincts are inadequate because contemporary Western culture no longer allows individuals to experience the overpowering force of sexual desire in its original form. This disconnection fosters inner conflict, as the individual perceives themselves to be subordinated to a force they can neither fully integrate nor ignore.

From a biological perspective, however, Federn conceded that Tausk's position held merit. In earlier unicellular life forms, no real distinction existed between individual development and species propagation. In metazoans, part of the organism serves for individual maturation, while another part is reserved for reproduction. Thus, the sexual organs, once integral to the original cell, have become separate systems, and the individual can be viewed as merely an organ serving the reproductive function.

Sachs proposed a terminological revision. Rather than relying on the problematic and often morally charged terms *sadism* and *masochism*, he suggested using the concepts of "active and passive erotism of aggression." This shift aimed to clarify the phenomena under discussion without invoking unnecessary clinical or cultural connotations.

In his closing remarks, Tausk returned to the broader theoretical stakes of his talk. He reiterated that his goal had been to demonstrate how the concept of "ego instincts" could be illuminated through their opposition to sexual instincts. Psychologically, what appears in consciousness is merely a representation of biological dynamics. If Freud explained repression through the vicissitudes of species preservation, then it is again a matter of contrasting two representations: that of the species and that of the individual. The child's desire to appropriate everything for the self is met with demands from the species for sacrifice and renunciation, leading to inner conflict. Addressing the association between repression and constipation, Tausk underscored that both groups of instincts may employ the same somatic organs, differing only in the sequence of their dominance—a notion reminiscent of Rank's hierarchical theory of the instincts. Federn's remark that the individual functions as an "organ of the sexual organ" thus touches the crux of the issue: the human being must serve two opposing tendencies, thereby laying the groundwork for psychic contradiction and intrapsychic conflict.

Beyond the specific contributions of each discussant, this historical debate carried important theoretical and technical implications—particularly for Freud, Spielrein, and Jung. Freud, as noted earlier, briefly remarked—without elaboration—that the problem of masochism mirrored that of the death drive. Spielrein interpreted this as tacit validation of her own thesis. Nonetheless, Freud's conceptual framework ultimately diverged from hers. While Spielrein rooted repression in the ego-threatening destructiveness of sexuality, Freud maintained that it stemmed from ambivalence—an intrinsic duality of affect that underpins all psychic life. This key theoretical divergence would re-emerge in Freud's later writings, especially those concerning narcissism and the phylogenetic origins of repression. As Kerr (1993) has argued, Freud's reframing of these issues subtly served to minimize Spielrein's contributions while simultaneously discrediting Jung's broader influence.

Following the scientific session of March 27, 1912, in which Viktor Tausk was the speaker, Ernest Jones would later describe what he considered a notable and frequently cited confrontation between Tausk and Stekel. As I will demonstrate below, Jones (1955, p. 136) attributes the origins of this conflict only vaguely, stating that "for some reason, Tausk and Stekel disliked each other." However, as detailed elsewhere in this book, the beginnings of this animosity can be traced back to the Vienna Psychoanalytic Society meeting held on November 24, 1909, where Tausk presented his first paper to the Society, "Theory of knowledge and psychoanalysis." As argued earlier, Jones was unaware of what transpired at that meeting, including Stekel's own account of Tausk's reaction to his intervention to "save the situation" (Gutheil, 1950, p. 133). This lack of awareness—combined with the absence of any reference to that episode—explains both the vagueness and the chronological inaccuracy in Jones's attribution of the origins of the Stekel–Tausk conflict. Jones's knowledge of their animosity appears to have derived mainly from his reading of the correspondence between Freud and Ferenczi, as will be discussed shortly.

In the second volume of *The Life and Work of Sigmund Freud*, Jones (1955, p. 136) narrates an especially heated exchange between Tausk and Stekel during a session he dates to May 30, 1912. According to his account, the meeting was marked by "a very ugly scene" in which Tausk accused Stekel of being incapable of articulating a coherent sentence. In turn, Stekel allegedly retorted that not a single line written by Tausk would ever appear in the *Zentralblatt für Psychoanalyse*—the official organ of the International Psychoanalytic Association, of which Stekel was editor.

However, the fourth volume of the *Minutes of the Vienna Psychoanalytic Society* (Nunberg & Federn, 1975, p. vii) contains no record of a meeting on May 30, 1912. This discrepancy suggests that Jones's account may stem from a lapse of memory, a conflation of different events, or perhaps an undocumented informal gathering. A clarifying footnote in that same volume (Nunberg & Federn, 1975, p. 102) specifies that, at the end of the 1911–1912 working year, three additional meetings were held—on May 15, May 22, and May 29—but no minutes were preserved, nor do the *Zentralblatt* issues from that period provide reports of them.

Jones's reference to a session on May 30, therefore, does not align with the Society's documented calendar. Nonetheless, he appears to base his reconstruction, at least in part, on a letter from Freud to Ferenczi dated May 30, 1912 (Falzeder et al., 1994, p. 377), in which Freud wrote:

> The Society was closed yesterday, but will convene unofficially every other Wednesday, and, when Jones is here, it will hold its customary summer festival. Before Whitsun there was another ugly scene between

> Tausk, who is a wild beast, and Stekel, which had all kinds of epilogues as a consequence. Stekel has become negligent in attendance lately, evidently doesn't feel comfortable, and, since he is still in contact with Adler, surprises seem to me to be not out of the question. So, good and bad are mixing together.

This letter appears to be Jones's principal documentary source for his reconstruction. Yet, in the published biography, Jones limits himself to the imprecise assertion that "for some reason Stekel and Tausk were in open conflict," without substantiating this with other evidence. He writes:

> It happened that for some reason Stekel and Tausk hated each other, and at the last meeting of the session 1911–1912 (May 30, 1912) there was a very ugly scene between them. Now Freud, although he once designated him as a "wild beast," had a very high opinion of Tausk's capacity, and just then wanted him to supervise the reviewing department of the *Zentralblatt*, which had been sadly neglected [...] Stekel was at once up in arms and declared he would not allow a line from Tausk's pen to appear in his *Zentralblatt*. Freud reminded him that it was the official organ of the International Association and that such personal claims were out of place.
> (Jones, 1955, p. 136)

Jones's widely cited account thus rests exclusively on the Freud–Ferenczi correspondence and not on other relevant documentary sources—namely, the *Minutes of the Vienna Psychoanalytic Society* (Nunberg & Federn, 1967) and Stekel's autobiography (Gutheil, 1950), both of which were available to Eissler and informed his far more meticulous reconstruction of the Stekel–Tausk conflict. From a historiographical standpoint, the methodological contrast is stark: whereas Eissler evidences a scrupulous analysis of all extant sources, Jones's treatment remains selective and imprecise.

Adding to this contentious history, Tausk had previously accused Stekel of inventing clinical cases to bolster his theoretical claims (Makari, 2008, p. 266). Stekel, in turn, threatened to resign from the International Psychoanalytic Association unless the insult was formally condemned. Freud, seeking to defuse the conflict, advised Tausk to avoid personal attacks (Gutheil, 1950, p. 142). Yet he himself remained critical of Stekel's editorial practices—particularly what he saw as an abuse of authority in threatening to exclude Tausk from the *Zentralblatt*.

When Stekel refused to step down as editor, Freud appealed directly to the publishers, the Bergmanns, requesting his removal. This, however, proved unfeasible because of substantial financial commitments (Stanton, 1991; Kerr, 1993). In a strategic countermove, Freud urged the journal's subscribers to cancel their subscriptions. The community largely complied, and within a year the *Zentralblatt für Psychoanalyse* ceased publication (Jones, 1955, p. 137).

These events precipitated Stekel's resignation from the Vienna Psychoanalytic Society, though he made one final—albeit unsuccessful—attempt to reconcile with Freud before leaving the movement altogether (Gay, 1988).

In the wake of this series of destabilizing events—including Adler's defection, Stekel's resignation, and the growing estrangement of Jung—Ernest Jones met with Sándor Ferenczi in Vienna in July 1912. In response to these internal fractures, Jones proposed the formation of a *Secret Committee* to preserve the coherence and continuity of psychoanalysis. After discussing the proposal with Rank, they presented it to Freud, who welcomed it with enthusiasm (Grosskurth, 1986).

Soon thereafter, the annual Psychoanalytic Congress scheduled for September was canceled. Jung, still serving as President of the IPA, was preparing to travel to the United States to deliver a highly anticipated series of lectures at Fordham University in New York. On October 9, the first post-summer meeting of the IPA convened, and at Freud's initiative, it was decided to create a *Review Committee.* This body would critically evaluate newly published psychoanalytic works—especially those appearing in the *Jahrbuch*—and publish the reviews in the *Internationale Zeitschrift für Ärztliche Psychoanalyse.* Accordingly, *Jahrbuch, 4*—excluding contributions by Freud and Jones—was examined in the first issues of the *Zeitschrift*. For example, in *Zeitschrift, 1*(*1*), Viktor Tausk reviewed articles by Jan Władysław Nelken and Shaina (Scheina/Jenny) Grebelskaja, while in issue *1*(*2*) Eduard Hitschmann critiqued works by Otto Rank and Herbert Silberer. Paul Federn was assigned to review Sabina Spielrein's essay, and Rudolf Reitler—often cited as the second psychoanalyst in history—evaluated a contribution by Eugen Bleuler (Freud & Jung, 1974/1978).

Before resuming the main narrative, it is worth tracing brief portraits of Nelken and Grebelskaja, whose work Tausk reviewed (Tausk, 1913a, 1913b). Jan Władysław Nelken (1878–1940) was perhaps the most original and promising figure of the first generation of Polish psychoanalysts. Employed in Piltz's clinic from 1908, he became an assistant the following year at Zürich's renowned Burghölzli Hospital, where he quickly earned the esteem of Eugen Bleuler and, above all, Carl Gustav Jung, with whom he collaborated on pioneering research into the links between mythology and fantasy in schizophrenia. During the interwar years, Nelken served as a military colonel doctor in the Kozielsk camp and was murdered by the Soviets at Katyń in 1940 (Katyń Foundation, 2025; Dybel, 2020, p. 147).

Shaina (Scheina/Jenny) Grebelskaja (1886–?) likewise trained with Bleuler and Jung at the Burghölzli, where she also served as a summer assistant. In 1912, she earned her medical degree with a dissertation on the psychological analysis of a paranoid patient—a study highly valued by Tausk (1913b) for its nuanced exploration of repressed homosexual desire in paranoia, lending empirical support to Freud's thesis on the subject. A close friend of Sabina Spielrein (Launer, 2014, p. 112), Grebelskaja returned to Russia later that same year to practice as a gynecologist in Odessa; after that, her professional and personal path fades entirely from the historical record (Psychoanalytikerinnen in der Schweiz, 2025).

Although their life stories diverged, Nelken and Grebelskaja shared a formative chapter at the Burghölzli—a crucible that, in my view, left a lasting mark on the way each approached and practiced psychoanalysis. With this context in place, it is now time to return to the main narrative: by late October 1912, Lou Andreas-Salomé had already begun to take notice of Viktor Tausk. On October 30, during a meeting of the Vienna Psychoanalytic Society held at the College of Physicians, she described him in her diary as a "stubborn blond," acknowledging that some of his remarks stirred resistance in her. At that same meeting, Sigmund Freud served as the speaker, delivering a presentation titled "Communication about a case, combined with some polemical observations." According to a footnote in the fourth volume of the *Minutes*, this was the first occasion on which "this famous woman"—a clear reference to Andreas-Salomé—is mentioned as a guest in the official records; in subsequent entries, she would appear simply as "Lou" (Nunberg & Federn, 1975, p. 108). At the time, she was living in Vienna with her companion, the German writer and actress Ellen Delp (1890–1990), and intended to pursue formal psychoanalytic training (Peters, 1962/1995).

Freud's presentation on that occasion, blending clinical material with theoretical critique, centered on the castration complex and its relation to neurosis and character formation—an area he emphasized was still in need of deeper exploration. He observed that the girl desires the penis when she sees another person possess an organ of apparent power and value. This sexual envy later resurfaces as envy of the mother's more mature bodily form. Freud framed sexual envy as a narcissistic phenomenon, arising at a point when no clear distinction exists between ego and sexual instincts.

As noted in a footnote by the editors of the *Minutes*, Freud's contribution stood out in its clarity and force. "One is, so to say, relieved to hear, after quite a few rather sterile discussions, these simple and clear words," they remarked. "As if with a spotlight, they illuminate Adler's error and show, in an unambiguous manner, the vicissitudes of the castration complex in the man, and of penis envy in the woman" (Nunberg & Federn, 1975, p. 112). Furthermore, the editors added that Freud's remarks conveyed a striking insight not recorded elsewhere: that neurotic doubting is, among other things, the perception of one's own ambivalence, and that feelings of inferiority can be understood as reactions to the perception of one's own inhibitions.

To bring this remarkable session to a close, it is worth underscoring the contribution of Viktor Tausk himself—the central figure of this study. At the same time, those wishing to explore the discussion in greater depth may consult the full record in the *Minutes* (Nunberg & Federn, 1975, pp. 108–112), where Freud's clinical reflections and his critiques of Adlerian theory—particularly with regard to the "masculine protest"—are further elaborated. Responding directly to these ideas, Tausk commented that Adler had treated inferiority as though it were merely the psychic representation of a somatic condition, while paradoxically basing the masculine protest on something psychic: a reactive process. On Adler's general cultural commentary, Tausk remarked that it remained largely commonplace. Drawing from his clinical experience, Tausk identified specific phenomena that, in his view, revealed the workings of the castration complex. He noted that anesthesia of the penis during coition could serve as one such manifestation, and that exhibitionistic behavior often pointed in the same direction. In one case, a patient was unable to engage in sexual intercourse unless he could visually observe the act himself. In another, excessive urination—polyuria—was interpreted as an unconscious effort to reassure oneself of the continued presence of the penis.

Just days after the October 30 meeting, another session of the Vienna Psychoanalytic Society was held on November 6, 1912. On this occasion, the speaker was Isidor Sadger, who presented a paper titled "On the sadomasochistic complex." Lou Andreas-Salomé was again in attendance as a guest, and the emotionally charged atmosphere did not escape her attention. In her diary, she registered a growing sense of unease—further evidence of the mounting tension she perceived between Freud and Jung. Coming so soon after the previous meeting, this session offered Andreas-Salomé a deeper glimpse into both the scientific dynamics and the underlying interpersonal strains within the Society.

During that session, Andreas-Salomé observed how Freud, with characteristic understated irony, questioned the conceptual necessity of the "complex"—a term increasingly central to Jung's theoretical edifice. He likened the elevation of the concept within psychoanalysis to the deification of Dionysus, who, as he wryly remarked, had attained divine status solely by virtue of being the son of Zeus. The analogy, though veiled, subtly cast Freud himself in a quasi-divine role, with Jung as the over-elevated offspring. Viktor Tausk, who arrived late to the meeting, is noted to have smiled ironically at Freud's comment, suggesting both his appreciation of the rhetorical gesture and his alignment with Freud's implicit critique (Andreas-Salomé, 1958/1984).

On November 6, 1912, Lou Andreas-Salomé also recorded in her journal that she had attended a lecture by Tausk designed to introduce the essential principles of Freudian theory. The presentation, held at the *Institut für Therapie nervöser Geiststörungen* under the direction of Karl Weiss (1879–?), drew an audience of approximately 40 people. Of Weiss, only a few details are known: he was a neurologist and psychoanalyst, born in Reichenberg (Bohemia, now Liberec, Czech Republic), though both the date and place of his death remain uncertain (Freud Museum, n.d.). From Andreas-Salomé's account, Tausk emerged as an intellectually brilliant and rhetorically gifted figure—marked, however, by an excessive deference toward Freud and a correspondingly sharp, even dismissive tone when speaking of Adler. That same evening, after the meeting of the Vienna Psychoanalytic Society already mentioned—at which Sadger, as noted earlier, presented his paper "On the sadomasochistic complex," a theme to which he was deeply devoted—Andreas-Salomé joined Tausk and Federn for a walk. During their conversation, the topic of Adler resurfaced: Tausk remained steadfast in his criticisms, while Federn adopted a more balanced and nuanced stance (Andreas-Salomé, 1958/1984).

One week later, on November 13, 1912, the Vienna Psychoanalytic Society reconvened for a second discussion of Sadger's previously introduced paper, "On the sadomasochistic complex." On this occasion, Tausk offered a particularly incisive intervention. He argued that what had been demonstrated thus far was merely that the erotogenic zones are employed in a sadomasochistic fashion—but not where sadism itself originates. Nor had it been explained, he pointed out, why urethral and muscular erotism should bear a special relevance to such configurations, or under what specific conditions an individual with sensitive skin might develop into a sadomasochist. "What has been shown," Tausk stated, "is only that all the experiences from childhood that were mentioned are later made use of in a certain sense; the question is, why?" (Nunberg & Federn, 1975, p. 118). This question, however, remained unanswered in that evening's scientific exchange, revealing both the richness and the unresolved tensions within Sadger's conceptualization.

Two weeks later, on November 27, 1912, Tausk presented a paper of his own before the Society, titled "Two contributions to the psychoanalysis of artistic inhibitions"—a work that would be published the following year. In it, he presented two clinical cases—one of a painter and one of a writer—to illustrate how artistic inhibition results from the heightened intensity of a drive or drive component, fixated in an infantile manner on specific persons or situations. When such a fixation was triggered, the libido could no longer be displaced; instead, the drive compulsively sought its specific mode of satisfaction, resulting in inhibition. The main point of contention concerned Tausk's treatment of narcissism. Freud responded with marked severity, reproaching Tausk for publishing prematurely and without sufficient theoretical rigor. Andreas-Salomé, reflecting on these events, conceived the tension between them as a clash of two formidable intellects—those of Freud and Tausk (Andreas-Salomé, 1958/1984). Yet if this were not enough, the year culminated in a particularly charged moment. On Saturday, December 14, 1912, during Freud's course on the psychoanalytic treatment of neuroses, Tausk delivered a pointed critique of the psychoanalytic method itself. He argued that by fragmenting the analysand's psychic material, psychoanalysis risked alienating the subject and impeding the formation of a coherent, unified sense of self. According to Lou Andreas-Salomé, the only attendee who appeared to share Tausk's unease was Viktor Emil Freiherr von Gebsattel (1883–1976), philosopher and participant in the Weimar Congress. Gebsattel had previously articulated similar concerns in his essay "Der Einzelne und der Zuschauer: Untersuchung zur Psychologie und Pathologie des Triebes nach Beachtung" [The individual and the spectator: An inquiry into the psychology and pathology of the drive for attention] (Gebsattel, 1912), where he examined the conflict between the subject's inner unity and the objectifying gaze of psychological interpretation—an anxiety that resonates profoundly with Tausk's critique.

Tausk argued that psychoanalysis, while aspiring to scientific legitimacy, paradoxically aimed to access the totality of the subject's inner life—an aim inherently resistant to analytic dissection. He proposed that if psychoanalysis were reconceived as a method capable of grasping the full breadth of the analysand's being, rather than reducing it to fragmented drives or symptoms, its therapeutic potential could be fundamentally redefined.

At the heart of this critique was the enduring problem of transference. Freud had initially addressed the concept in 1905 in "Fragment of an analysis of a case of hysteria (the Dora case)," where he acknowledged that transference created both resistance and opportunity—it reenacted childhood conflicts within the analytic setting, impeding their direct retrieval into consciousness (Freud, 1905b/1978b). In his 1912 essay "The dynamics of transference," Freud developed the concept further, concluding that a skillful handling of transference was not an obstacle but the cornerstone of therapeutic success (Freud, 1912a/1980c). The analytic setting, by allowing the return of the original infantile neurosis in the form of a "transference neurosis," created the very conditions necessary for transformation. As Freud famously observed, "no one can be judged *in absentia* or in effigie." Only through the lived, present-tense engagement with transference could a genuine working-through be achieved (Freud, 1914c/1980f). Elsewhere in *The Freud Journal* (Andreas-Salomé, 1958/1984), Lou refers to an essay on Spinoza (Spinoza-Dialog), originally written by Tausk in 1907 and subsequently revised by him years later. Notably, eight years after its initial composition, Tausk added the following reflection:

"Every word in this dialogue has retained its validity for me to the present" ("*Jedes Wort in dieser Schrift gilt mir auch heute noch*"). It is "a spoken scene between the *exalted Spinoza* and a man known for me" ("*Eine gesprochene Szene zwischen dem* Erhabenen Spinoza *und einem mir bekannten Menschen*") (Tausk, 1915, as cited in Eissler, 1983, p. 20).

The unnamed interlocutor to whom Tausk alludes is, in fact, none other than himself—a subtle yet revealing testament to the profound influence that Spinoza exerted on his intellectual development.

This influence becomes particularly evident in Tausk's philosophical manuscript "Theory of knowledge and psychoanalysis," discovered among Lou Andreas-Salomé's personal papers after her death in 1937. As previously noted in this book, it is in *The Freud Journal* (Andreas-Salomé, 1958/1984) that Lou first mentions this manuscript, emphasizing its importance in shaping Tausk's intellectual development. At the time of her reference, however, nothing further was known about the work or its content beyond Andreas-Salomé's brief remarks in her diary. Nearly a decade later, in 1967, the same manuscript unexpectedly resurfaced in *Minutes of the Vienna Psychoanalytic*

Society as the record of Tausk's first formal presentation to the Society, delivered on November 24, 1909 (Nunberg & Federn, 1967, pp. 328–337). The circumstances through which the text—originally found among Andreas-Salomé's effects—came to be included in the official archival volume remain uncertain. Nonetheless, its publication marked a pivotal moment in the historiography of Tausk's contributions to psychoanalysis. Selected passages from this presentation were later quoted by Kurt R. Eissler in *Victor Tausk's Suicide* (1983), further drawing attention to this early and philosophically ambitious work.

For Andreas-Salomé, one of the manuscript's most meaningful contributions lies in its elucidation of the true philosophical origin of the term "representation." Although she had initially believed this concept to be uniquely Tausk's, she later came to recognize its Spinozist lineage—aptly describing Spinoza as "the philosopher of psychoanalysis." In her view, the idea that both physical and spiritual phenomena are to be understood as "representations" can be traced directly back to Spinoza. This conception departs from classical psycho-physical parallelism, asserting instead that mind and body are but two aspects of a single ontological substance (Andreas-Salomé, 1958/1984).

Another Spinozist notion that left a deep imprint on Tausk's worldview was the conviction that human beings are, in essence, unfree—governed by necessity and determined by causality. However, Spinoza holds that through knowledge and the use of reason, the individual may attain a form of limited freedom. This cognitive liberation allows the subject to rise above external obligations and constraints, while simultaneously gaining insight into the inner determinism that governs their own nature. Moreover, in Spinoza's philosophy, every entity, insofar as it exists, strives to persevere in its being—a striving he termed *conatus*, the very essence of each thing. The highest goal of existence, then, is the preservation of that existence. Thus, for Spinoza—and, by extension, for Tausk—desire becomes the truest expression of the human condition: a ceaseless yearning by which the subject seeks to transcend finitude and attain a form of eternity (Marías, 1941/1970).

At the outset of 1913, specifically on Wednesday, January 11, a fervent debate took place between Tausk and Seif concerning Jung. Among the attendees were Rank, Hitschmann, and several others who remained neutral observers. According to Andreas-Salomé, Tausk delivered an exceptionally compelling intervention, which, in turn, elicited an undercurrent of unease and jealousy from Rank.

Leonhard Seif (1866–1949), a neurologist from Munich and director of the city's Psychoanalytic Association, had founded the Munich Psychoanalytic Association in 1912, having previously been a member of Freud's Zürich group established in 1907 (Kerr, 1993). In her journal, Lou also recounts her collaborative work with Tausk during the early days of February 1913. Together, they worked on a critique of James Jackson Putnam (1846–1918), professor of neurology at Harvard Medical School in Boston. Putnam had at first rejected psychoanalysis, yet eventually became one of its most devoted supporters in the United States. At the same time, Tausk and Andreas-Salomé collaborated on the preparation of the second lecture in a course on anxiety that Tausk was then delivering.

Regarding the critique of Putnam, Lou notes that during its presentation before the Vienna Psychoanalytic Association, Freud—who held Putnam in great esteem—abruptly silenced Tausk. The gesture caused visible discomfort among those present. Later, after venting his frustration to Federn, Tausk could only watch in dismay as a rumor spread that he had privately sought Freud's permission to criticize Putnam's work. The next day, Lou engaged Freud in a long conversation about the incident. While she acknowledged the sincerity of his convictions and understood the reasoning behind his anger, she nonetheless concluded that Freud found it difficult to tolerate another person who was both assertive and intellectually independent. Such individuals, she observed, challenged Freud's self-image as a solitary pioneer and, in doing so, risked sowing the seeds of future dissent (Andreas-Salomé, 1958/1984).

Among Putnam's contributions was an essay published in *Imago* titled "The role of philosophical views and training in the further development of the psychoanalytic movement" (Putnam, 1912; Nunberg & Federn, 1975, p. 162), originally presented at the Weimar Congress. The paper was soon met with criticism from Sándor Ferenczi in "Philosophy and psychoanalysis" (Ferenczi, 1912/1981b), followed by Tausk's own response discussed above.

Ferenczi, while acknowledging the legitimate influence that other sciences might exert on psychoanalysis, firmly rejected Putnam's thesis that psychoanalysis must be subsumed within a broader philosophical system. For Ferenczi, psychoanalysis constituted a scientific discipline in its own right. He likened science to an enterprise that produces new values, whereas philosophy, in contrast, was viewed as a worldview—an interpretive framework that, based on current knowledge, may occasionally help guide future intellectual endeavors (Ferenczi, 1912/1981b).

On March 12, 1913, Lou Andreas-Salomé attended Viktor Tausk's lecture "The father problem" at the Vienna Psychoanalytic Society. After the session, she met Freud, who had been waiting for her outside. During their walk, Freud made a troubling admission: he had recognized in Tausk's lecture ideas strikingly similar to his own. Yet, despite this resemblance, he dismissed the work. Freud argued that it failed to link psychoanalytic theory convincingly with clinical experience—particularly with the neuroses. He also objected to Tausk's reliance on Johann Jakob Bachofen (1815–1887), the Swiss historian of law, philosopher, and theorist of matriarchy. Freud maintained that this dependence distorted the analysis by overlooking the central psychoanalytic function of the incest prohibition, which, he insisted, found clearer expression within a patriarchal framework. Two days later, the topic resurfaced during a private conversation at Freud's home (Andreas-Salomé, 1958/1984).

Before turning to Freud's pointed criticisms, it is worth outlining the principal arguments presented by Tausk in that lecture. Taking for granted the fundamental role of the father complex as both the vehicle and content of neurosis, Tausk set out to examine the broader implications of this complex—not only in individual psychic life but also in the structure of society itself. To pursue this aim, he temporarily abstracted the father complex from its clinical setting in order to trace its function in the development of cultural institutions.

Tausk began by noting that the paternal figure does not occupy the same symbolic authority in all civilizations. He drew on Bachofen's reconstruction of matriarchal societies—derived from juridical, religious, and mythological sources as well as symbolic rituals and customs—as a counterpoint to the later patriarchal systems (Bachofen, 1861). In the Roman patriarchate, for instance, the father's omnipotence was paradoxically accompanied by a prohibition against incest with his daughter, even while he retained power over his children's lives and liberty. Tausk interpreted this as evidence that the patriarchal structure evolved in tandem with the renunciation of incest—a renunciation that may have originated biologically, due to the presumed degenerative effects of incest—and was ultimately institutionalized through social mechanisms such as marriage, virginity guarantees, and the control of female sexuality.

This renunciation, Tausk argued, also gave rise to male dominion and the separation of sons from access to the same women, thereby laying the foundation of patriarchal order. He suggested that early incest prohibitions may have initially targeted sodomy, with patricide prohibited to protect paternal authority, while the killing of sons—eventually symbolically replaced by castration—was tolerated. Circumcision, in this view, remains a cultural residue of such symbolic acts.

From here, Tausk linked the father complex to ambivalent affective structures in the son, whose love for the father is interwoven with rebellion and unconscious hatred—born of restrictions, displaced desire for the mother, and unresolved homosexual fixations. He maintained that it is this ambivalence that facilitates both the formation of neurosis and the sublimation necessary for cultural development. Indeed, society itself, Tausk concluded, rests on the symbolic figure of the father. Even religion, he suggested, arises through a displacement of this ambivalence, whereby the hostile father is transformed into a divine figure through identification and sublimated love. Ultimately, Tausk proposed that the father complex was not merely a personal psychic structure but the very foundation upon which society, culture, and interpersonal bonds are built.

Despite the philosophical and anthropological richness of this account, it drew sustained criticism from Freud and other members of the Society. According to the meeting records, Freud found that Tausk failed to meet the central requirement of the topic: to demonstrate how neurosis derives from the father complex, and how that same complex in turn influences society (Nunberg & Federn, 1975, p. 180). Freud pointed out that the lecture lacked crucial components—most notably, an explanation of the transition from matriarchy to the family structure and the psychological origins of the incest taboo. He dismissed the biological account as untenable and noted the paradox that incest, far from being universally condemned, had at times held sacred or legal status among certain advanced civilizations. He further emphasized that incest prohibitions predate the institution of marriage, and argued that the topic of virginity within patriarchal frameworks warranted its own focused treatment. Freud concluded by remarking that he would soon present his own views on these issues—an allusion to *Totem and Taboo* (Freud, 1913/1980e).

Other commentators echoed Freud's objections. Sachs and Federn challenged the empirical foundations of Bachofen's theory, observing that its evidentiary basis might represent psychic wishes rather than historical realities. Federn also questioned the logic of deriving incest prohibition from totemic traditions, suggesting instead that the patriarchal family had to exist prior to such taboos. Moreover, he found that Tausk failed to adequately explain the psychic necessity of incest prohibition or convincingly relate it to the onset of neurosis.

Rank criticized the order in which Tausk presented his ideas, arguing that he should have begun with clinical neurosis, then turned to the psychic father complex, and only afterward to cultural developments. As it stood, Rank observed, the lecture devoted too much attention to cultural history, while treating neurosis merely as an afterthought. Hitschmann offered the sharpest critique, accusing Tausk of confusing the central issue. In his view, the presentation had little relevance either to neurosis or to the analytic understanding of the father complex.

In sum, while Tausk's lecture ambitiously sought to integrate psychoanalysis, cultural anthropology, and social theory, it ultimately failed to persuade his analytic peers—most notably Freud himself. Their criticisms reveal the epistemological tensions between psychoanalysis as a clinical science rooted in the treatment of neuroses and its broader application to the interpretation of culture and civilization.

Having established this, I now return to examine how the figure of Viktor Tausk increasingly came to occupy a central place in Lou Andreas-Salomé's intellectual world. Throughout her intimate impressions collected in *The Freud Journal* (Andreas-Salomé, 1958/1984), Lou returns repeatedly to the subject of Tausk—a testament to the intensity and complexity of their evolving relationship. Of particular interest are the entries spanning August 21 to September 5, 1913, following Lou's return to Vienna in the company of Rainer Maria Rilke, after an extended absence that had begun in April.

In her autobiographical notes, Lou offers a psychologically penetrating observation: she identifies in Tausk an irresistible drive to position himself in the role of the son—and, by extension, to harbor resentment toward the father. This dynamic, she suggests, may well explain a recurrent inhibition in Tausk's intellectual output. While he possessed striking analytical and synthetic gifts, these capacities—which had shone brightly in the context of philosophical exchange—seemed to falter when he ventured into domains closely associated with Freud's own theoretical preoccupations.

Indeed, what Lou perceived was not a lack of talent, but rather an unconscious entanglement: as Tausk drew nearer to the intellectual territory already mapped by Freud, his thinking appeared to grow constrained, as though the father's presence simultaneously inspired and paralyzed him (Andreas-Salomé, 1958/1984). The more he strove to define his own position within the psychoanalytic field, the more difficult it became to disentangle his originality from the gravitational pull of Freud's authority. Even in his efforts to articulate independent theoretical perspectives, Tausk remained psychically tethered to Freud's influence—both invigorated and eclipsed by it.

Admitting all that has been previously stated, the Freud–Tausk conflict came to be inscribed within a neurotic struggle deeply marked by unresolved filial–paternal tensions—a struggle that, for both men, offered no clear path to resolution. In his pursuit of recognition, Tausk gradually assumed the psychic position of a son in relation to the master, which bound him in a contradictory and tormenting web of admiration, longing, and rivalry. In this context, Eissler (1971) insightfully observed that "in the end, she [Lou Andreas-Salomé] was already recognizing that this man [Tausk] was irreconcilably divided in himself and destined for doom. She discovered that, even in his thinking processes, he was entangled in an insoluble conflict about Freud" (p. 41).

Her perception underscored not only the intensity of Tausk's inner turmoil, but also the tragic impasse at the heart of his bond with Freud—an impasse that neither intellect nor affection could resolve.

Lou Andreas-Salomé consistently returned to this dynamic in her *The Freud Journal* (Andreas-Salomé, 1958/1984). She noted with particular poignancy the urgency with which Tausk sought analysis from Freud—a need propelled by an irreconcilable constellation of affective and intellectual conflicts. Freud, for his part, was not immune to the emotional strain of their relationship. In a moment of frustrated clarity, he is said to have referred to Tausk as a *Raubtier*—a predatory animal—while Tausk, paradoxically, sought safety and recognition in Freud's paternal embrace.

Yet such moments of affective proximity were fleeting. According to Lou, Tausk was afflicted by a deep and relentless yearning for maternal love—a craving so fundamental that, had she been capable of fulfilling it, the grief and disquiet that tormented his soul might have found some measure of relief. In *The Freud Journal* (Andreas-Salomé, 1958/1984, p. 186), she refers to him with a poignant expression of intimate kinship: "*Der Kampf der menschlichen Kreatur. Brudertier, Du*" ["The struggle of the human creature. Brother animal, you"]. This phrase encapsulates both the tenderness and raw vulnerability she perceived in him—a creature suspended between intellect and instinct, between sublimation and bodily longing. That Lou chose to describe Tausk in such terms signals, in my view, the particular form of intimacy she was willing to offer: a sublimated bond, rich in emotional meaning yet removed from physical or sexual expression. It is doubtful, however, that Tausk experienced this boundary in the same way. For a man so tormented by inner conflict, Lou's affective distance may well have constituted a narcissistic wound—an implicit rejection that pierced the core of his embodied self. The animal—the vulnerable, desiring creature that Tausk represented—remained excluded from the realm of sexual *jouissance*. The boundaries of the body, and the shared erotic space he longed for, would never be crossed between them—an absence that, for Tausk, must have cut deeply.

Eissler (1971, p. 42), however, offers a markedly different reading. He laments that Paul Roazen, in titling his book *Brother Animal* (Roazen, 1969), extracted Lou's phrase from its context and, in doing so, distorted its meaning:

> It is a part of this final phrase that he used as the title of his book, thereby transforming a beautiful, superbly touching epilogue into something offensively coarse, if not downright vulgar. What he has done is to tear these final words out of context and use the English translation, which implies the very opposite of the German original, thus converting a poetic expression of the greatest feeling of closeness between a man and a woman into a repellent epithet, which Roazen then employs to characterize a nonexistent rivalry between two men.

While Eissler's critique underscores the poetic and affective depth of Lou's phrase, it also highlights how easily the subtle interplay of meaning—especially when filtered through translation—can be lost or even inverted. In truth, the relationship between Lou Andreas-Salomé and Viktor Tausk was grounded in an emotionally and intellectually intense bond, shaped by deep currents of transference and unfulfilled maternal longing. Yet this relationship unfolded not in isolation, but in resonance with the broader tensions of the early psychoanalytic movement.

Tausk's attachment to Lou—and his simultaneous identification with Freud as a father figure—formed part of a more intricate drama, one in which personal longing, theoretical allegiance, and institutional positioning became inextricably entangled. His inner conflict, marked by unresolved filial dynamics, would find its tragic echo in the shifting allegiances, silent exclusions, and emotional ruptures that came to define the psychoanalytic community itself.

From a very different vantage point—namely, the expansion and institutional consolidation of psychoanalysis—another episode of lasting consequence was the Fourth International Psychoanalytic Congress, held in Munich on September 7 and 8, 1913. At this gathering, the Budapest

Psychoanalytic Association was formally accepted as an affiliate of the IPA, signaling a promising new stage in the movement's international reach. Yet the moment of collective celebration was quickly clouded by the fraught re-election of Carl Gustav Jung as President of the IPA. While Jung retained the post, his re-election was far from unanimous: of the 52 eligible voting members, 22 abstained, including Sándor Ferenczi—an abstention that prompted Jung to furiously brand him a traitor.

Lou noted Jung's conduct with some dismay, describing it as unusually harsh—a demeanor that visibly wounded Freud. Even Tausk's steadfast loyalty and defense of Freud at the congress could not alleviate the founder's sense of betrayal. Although Freud had, on occasion, voiced confidence in Tausk's potential as a future leader of the movement, he hesitated to act on such thoughts. The danger, Freud admitted, lay in Tausk's formidable intellect coupled with an unstable temperament; he once remarked that Tausk knew "how to bark and to bite." The Munich Congress thus marked a pivotal juncture in Tausk's position within the psychoanalytic establishment. In response to the controversies surrounding Jung's leadership, Tausk initiated a critical discussion about the IPA's future direction—a move that led, however, not to greater clarity but to his abrupt withdrawal from the congress. The immediate catalyst appears to have been an act of retaliation by Jung, who severely limited the time allocated for the presentation of a paper Tausk had co-authored with Lou Andreas-Salomé: "The psychological and pathological significance of narcissism."

The emotional toll of that episode would linger for years. In a letter to Lou dated March 26, 1919—six years after the Munich events—Tausk spoke of the enduring solitude he had felt ever since, asking whether she knew of any woman with whom he might share the remainder of his life. The letter, poignant and resigned, marked the final rupture of their intimate connection (Livingstone, 1984/1990). Its aftermath extended even into Tausk's analytic work: during his later treatment with Helene Deutsch, he confessed a profound and paradoxical revulsion toward Lou—particularly toward her breasts—which he said provoked in him a visceral sensation of nausea (Roazen, 1992, p. 163). This strange inversion of love into disgust may well have reflected the unresolved entanglement between maternal longing and narcissistic injury—a dialectic that haunted Tausk's emotional life as much as it shaped his theoretical contributions and institutional fate.

Freud, in his reflective essay "On the history of the psychoanalytic movement" (Freud, 1914a/1979d), where he retraces the origins and evolution of his own creation—the psychoanalytic movement—later condemned Jung's conduct at the Munich Congress as both inappropriate and inconsiderate, particularly his decision to curtail speakers' allotted time in favor of extended discussion. The incident left a lasting impression on Max Eitingon (1881–1943), who would later found the Berlin Psychoanalytic Polyclinic; so disheartened was he by the proceedings that he even proposed dissolving the IPA altogether.

Despite these setbacks, Tausk remained intellectually active and productive. In the same year, he published several noteworthy articles, including "Compensation as a means of discounting the motive of repression" (Tausk, 1913c/1983a), "Depiction of the dreamer's situation within the dream" (Tausk, 1913d/1983a), and "A contribution to the psychology of child sexuality" (Tausk, 1913e/1983a). The second of these essays, originally titled "Darstellung der Lage des Träumers im Traum," appeared in 1913 in *Internationale Zeitschrift für Psychoanalyse, 1*, 378. This article is included in the Spanish edition of Tausk's collected works (Tausk, 1983a), published by Gedisa, yet it is absent from the English-language compilation (Roazen, 2017a). Whether this omission also occurs in the French, Italian, or German collections remains unclear, as I have not had access to those editions. What I can confirm, having compared the Spanish and English compilations, is that both include different selections of Tausk's writings, without offering any editorial rationale for their criteria.

To return to the main thread of my narrative—after this brief editorial aside, which I trust the reader will forgive—the controversy with Jung continued. In the *Internationale Zeitschrift für Ärztliche Psychoanalyse*, Jung (1913) published a response titled "Eine Bemerkung zur Tauskschen Kritik der Nelkenschen Arbeit" [A remark on Tausk's critique of Nelken's work]. The paper addressed Tausk's review of an article by Jan Nelken, a promising figure of the first generation of Polish psychoanalysts, tragically lost in the Katyń massacre, whom I have referenced earlier in this book. Nelken's 1912 contribution to the *Jahrbuch für psychoanalytische und psychopathologische Forschungen*—"Analytische Beobachtungen über Phantasien eines Schizophrenen" [Analytical observations on the fantasies of a schizophrenic]—proposed striking parallels between schizophrenic fantasies and ancient cosmogonic myths, offering a provocative synthesis of psychopathology and mythopoetic imagination (Nelken, 1912).

Tausk's critical engagement with Nelken's article took the form of a review published the following year under the same title as Nelken's work, "Analytische Beobachtungen über Phantasien eines Schizophrenen" [Analytical observations on the fantasies of a schizophrenic] (Tausk, 1913a), in the *Internationale Zeitschrift für Psychoanalyse, 1*, 84–87. In that same issue, he also contributed a brief review of a separate case study by Shaina (Scheina/Jenny) Grebelskaja—whom I have likewise discussed earlier in this book—whose paper, "Psychologische Analyse eines Paranoiden" [Psychological analysis of a paranoid], presented a psychologically oriented account of paranoid dynamics. Tausk's response appeared immediately thereafter, under the title "Sch. Grebelskaja: Psychologische Analyse eines Paranoiden" [Sch. Grebelskaja: Psychological analysis of a paranoid patient] (Tausk, 1913b, p. 88), in that same journal.

Since these two reviews remain untranslated and exist only in their original German, I have cited them according to their original publication dates (1913). This differs from the practice followed for the remainder of Tausk's psychoanalytic writings, which are referenced here through the 1983 Spanish edition published by Gedisa, or, in certain instances, through the English edition edited by Paul Roazen. I note this distinction to clarify the citation method adopted throughout this book when referring to Tausk's technical works.

In June 1914, Tausk earned his doctorate in medicine, rekindling hopes for personal fulfillment and professional stability. Yet these aspirations were swiftly shattered by the outbreak of World War I on July 28, 1914, an event that, like for so many intellectuals of his generation, brought a profound rupture to the rhythms of his life and work. Before being conscripted into military service in August 1915—a duty that would last until the end of the war in November 1918, during which he served first as chief psychiatrist and later as neurologist—Tausk sought to counterbalance his growing sense of despair through sustained intellectual and creative engagement. It was during this period that he produced several significant papers, among them "Two homosexual dreams" (Tausk, 1914b/1983a), "A dream of numbers" (Tausk, 1914c/1983a), and "Short contributions to the interpretation of dreams" (Tausk, 1914d/1983a). Of these three articles, the first two—absent from the English edition of Tausk's collected works but included in the Spanish edition—were originally published in *Internationale Zeitschrift für Psychoanalyse, 2* (1914): "Zwei homosexuelle Träume" [Two homosexual dreams], pp. 36–39, and "Ein Zahlentraum" [A dream of numbers], pp. 39–41.

The third article, "Kleine Beiträge zur Traumdeutung" [Short contributions to dream interpretation: The use of clothes and colors in building up the dream picture], appeared in *Internationale Zeitschrift für Psychoanalyse, 2*, 464–466. In the English edition edited by Roazen (2017a, pp. 227–230), the title was adapted accordingly, while in the Spanish edition it was published under the abbreviated title "Short contributions to the interpretation of dreams." This editorial variation exemplifies the subtle yet consequential shifts that often accompany the translation and transmission of Tausk's work—an issue which, as I noted in Chapter 1, has undoubtedly shaped the reception and dissemination of his ideas within the international psychoanalytic community. A comprehensive examination of this process still awaits to be undertaken.

Before turning to the major milestones in Viktor Tausk's life, however, it is worth pausing to consider a lesser-known yet revealing text he published in 1914—one included in the English edition of his collected writings, though absent from the Spanish version. The essay, titled "Psychoanalysis of philosophy and psychoanalytic philosophy" (Roazen, 2017a, pp. 85–93), was originally published in German in the *Jahrbuch für psychoanalytische und psychopathologische Forschungen, 6*, 405–412, under the title "Psychoanalyse der Philosophie und psychoanalytische Philosophie" (Tausk, 1914a). Although concise, this early contribution is conceptually rich and offers a revealing glimpse into Tausk's reflections on the epistemological scope of psychoanalysis. Several of its key insights deserve particular attention.

Building on this introduction, Tausk examines the dynamic and often contentious intersection between psychoanalysis and philosophy. Despite the limited literature on the subject at the time, he remarks on the intensity of their overlap, particularly regarding psychological inquiry. He observes that philosophy had traditionally laid claim to the study of conscious psychology, while the boundaries of the unconscious remained undefined—producing a certain hesitation, even reluctance, in assigning particular ideas to one discipline or the other. Such hesitation, he suggests, often stems less from intellectual caution than from affective conflict.

Tausk further portrays the relationship between psychoanalysis and philosophy as unfolding along two interrelated paths. On the one hand, psychoanalysis has illuminated both the characterological underpinnings and the unconscious motivations of philosophers themselves; on the other, it has been applied to philosophical systems, revealing them as structured projections of intrapsychic dynamics. At the same time, psychoanalysis—especially in Freud's work—has yielded its own philosophical insights, offering conceptual tools that transcend the clinical domain and engage with fundamental questions of determinism, temporality, and the constitution of reality.

While the first two approaches represent applications of psychoanalytic insight to specific philosophical material—whether to the individual thinker or to the system of thought—the third stands apart as an original contribution of psychoanalysis to philosophy itself. These philosophical implications emerge chiefly from Freud's own theoretical developments, though references to them in other authors remain sparse and fragmentary. Whereas the first two lines of inquiry apply psychoanalytic understanding to external material, the third embodies psychoanalysis's intrinsic philosophical yield, of which Freud may be regarded as the principal exponent.

Following Freud's lead, the prevailing psychoanalytic view of the philosopher identifies a defining trait in the withdrawal of libidinal investment from the external world and its subsequent displacement onto the activity of thinking. Thought thereby becomes emotionally charged and assumes a reality comparable to that of external objects—an operation that aligns the philosopher, at a structural level, with the obsessional neurotic.

Tausk observes that Otto Rank and Hanns Sachs, in their early co-authored essay *Die Bedeutung der Psychoanalyse für die Geisteswissenschaften* [The significance of psychoanalysis for the humanities] (Rank & Sachs, 1913), propose a heuristic typology of philosophical figures grounded not in biographical detail or motivational psychology, but in configurations of libido. They distinguish three overarching tendencies: the intuitive or metaphysical type—exemplified by Plato, the mystics, and the speculative natural philosophers; the synthetic or empiricist type—represented by Auguste Comte (1798–1857), Herbert Spencer (1820–1903), and John Locke (1632–1704); and the analytic type—illustrated by Kant, Spinoza, René Descartes (1596–1650), and Hume. As Tausk clarifies, this classification concerns less the philosopher's individual psychology than the structural organization of philosophical systems viewed through the economy of libido.

Unlike Rank and Sachs (1913), authors such as Hitschmann and Freiherr von Winterstein avoid typological distinctions, attributing instead the genesis of philosophical thought to early infantile psychic constellations. Within this framework, philosophical systems appear as projections of inner psychic processes—often as *screen formations* organized around wish-fulfillment and rationalized *post hoc*. While the biographical substrate retains relevance, such systems also expose general laws of the psyche when subjected to proper analysis. Their epistemic content, insofar as it may be independently validated within other disciplines, remains beyond the scope of psychoanalytic critique.

Nietzsche is highlighted by both Hitschmann and Freiherr von Winterstein as a pivotal figure, one who—without the benefit of psychoanalytic theory—nonetheless grasped the affective undercurrents in philosophical thought.

Hitschmann, in particular, turns his attention to Schopenhauer, whom he regards as a proto-psychoanalytic thinker. In "Schopenhauer: Versuch einer Psychoanalyse des Philosophen" [Schopenhauer: An attempt at a psychoanalysis of the philosopher] (Hitschmann, 1913), he draws a compelling parallel between Schopenhauer's concept of the "will" and the Freudian unconscious, interpreting the philosopher's pervasive pessimism as the expression of a deep intrapsychic conflict—namely, the struggle between primal instinctual forces and the inhibiting functions of the ego. Schopenhauer's celebrated valorization of pure knowledge, dissociated from desire, is understood as a defense against instinctual life—a psychological strategy rooted in repression and conflict, not disinterest.

Tausk reports that, for Hitschmann, Schopenhauer's retreat into metaphysical negation, ascetic ideals, and mystical quietism signals masochistic tendencies shaped by unconscious guilt and a deficient sexual life. His metaphysics—defining the world as illusion—echoes melancholic symptomatology, suggesting a depressive denial of reality rooted in libidinal disappointment. Ultimately, Schopenhauer's philosophy is presented as the crystallization of a divided psychic structure, where ethical and metaphysical positions mirror unconscious repudiations of painful drives.

In Tausk's reconstruction, Alfred Freiherr von Winterstein, in his ambitious essay "Psychoanalytische Anmerkungen zur Geschichte der Philosophie" [Psychoanalytic notes on the history of philosophy] (Freiherr von Winterstein, 1913), undertakes the formidable task of applying psychoanalytic interpretation to the entire history of philosophy—though in doing so, he inevitably sacrifices a measure of structural clarity. Yet, as Tausk observes, Freiherr von Winterstein's readings remain firmly grounded in established psychoanalytic mechanisms, ultimately delineating the contours of a psychoanalytic philosophy that tends toward a realist–dualist epistemology. His distinctive contribution lies in selecting problems from within philosophy itself, approaching them not from a clinician's standpoint but from within the philosophical tradition, with full intellectual competence.

Freiherr von Winterstein emphasizes the philosopher's teachings as shaped by unconscious wishes, tracing how wish-fulfillment and intellectual elaboration intertwine. From Socrates (470–399 BCE) onward, he perceives a progressive devaluation of the external world and a compensatory turn inward. This withdrawal often assumes metaphysical form: Plato's *Ideas*, Kant's *noumenon*, and the Buddhist *nirvana* emerge as projections of unconscious needs to negate an intolerable reality. He explores how early libidinal configurations—such as voyeuristic and tactile pleasures—resurface in philosophical ideals of "knowing" or "merging" with the Absolute, as seen in the mystical ecstasies of Plotinus (204/205–270 CE), the founder of Neoplatonism. These moments of "insight," he suggests, represent regressions to primary sensory modalities and maternal fantasies. Philosophical *Eros*, in this context, becomes the longing to return to a timeless, pre-individuated state—an echo of the unconscious resistance to change and loss.

According to Freiherr von Winterstein, Plato's theory of Ideas constitutes not merely an intellectual doctrine but also a libidinal structure: the immutable, ideal images of the unconscious contrasted with the restless flux of empirical reality. The divine, likewise, appears as a projection of inner psychic authority—an idealized, omnipotent father-image infused with unconscious moral and sexual renunciations. Theories of emanation and creation, in turn, mirror distinct psychic constellations: emanation reflects narcissistic libidinal processes, while creation corresponds to symbolic gendered constructions of mind—as active and masculine—and matter—as passive and feminine.

From Tausk's perspective, Freiherr von Winterstein goes further still, correlating central philosophical doctrines—such as belief in pre-existence, transmigration of souls, and eternal return—with unconscious phenomena like *déjà vu*, libidinal displacement, and the cyclical rhythms of inner perception. His reading of Spinoza exemplifies this interpretive method: God becomes an extension of the father figure whose love cannot be directly claimed, leading to metaphysical compensations that veil unresolved oedipal longing.

In sum, Eduard Hitschmann and Alfred Freiherr von Winterstein converge on key psychoanalytic principles in their readings of philosophy—projection, wish-fulfillment, denial of reality, and the formative role of parental imagoes and drive conflicts. Where Hitschmann provides a detailed case study of Schopenhauer, Freiherr von Winterstein extends the analysis both historically and thematically, revealing how philosophical doctrines often function as rationalized derivatives of unconscious processes.

Tausk then turns his attention to philosophers who engaged with psychoanalysis itself, such as Paul Häberlin (1878–1960) and James Jackson Putnam, noting that both sought to preserve certain philosophical or moral assumptions and thereby to delimit the reach of psychoanalytic critique. Putnam, for example, defended a philosophy of life grounded in free agency, rejecting what he perceived as psychoanalytic determinism. Häberlin, in parallel, appealed to "deeper" cultural instincts transcending sexuality, thereby shielding core convictions from Freud's implications. In both cases, Tausk discerns a defensive maneuver: psychoanalysis is tolerated only insofar as it leaves intact pre-existing philosophical commitments.

Finally, Tausk offers a brief commentary on Jung's "Wandlungen und Symbole der Libido: Beiträge zur Entwicklungsgeschichte des Denkens" [Transformations and symbols of the libido: Contributions to the history of the development of thought] (Jung, 1912), a work analyzed more thoroughly by Ferenczi. He characterizes it as a synthetic generalization of psychoanalytic concepts—one that, however, incorporates elements foreign to psychoanalysis and ultimately departs from the Freudian metapsychological framework. In Tausk's view, such speculative systems, rather than continuing psychoanalytic inquiry, become legitimate objects of psychoanalytic interpretation in their own right.

In conclusion, Tausk reminds us that psychoanalysis itself—by its very principles—makes philosophical claims, especially concerning determinism and the temporal structure of psychic life. Freud's identification of distinct laws governing mental processes, above all the tension between the pleasure principle and the reality principle, implies a vision of ethical development grounded in biological and temporal adaptation. Through repression and symbolic elaboration, the pleasure principle transforms into the socially sustainable reality principle, suggesting that psychoanalytic mechanisms may indeed constitute the psychobiological foundation of philosophical and ethical reflection.

In parallel with the publication of his essay on psychoanalysis and philosophy, Tausk's intellectual activity continued to evolve. A noteworthy example is the oral presentation he delivered on December 30, 1914, before the Vienna Psychoanalytic Society (Nunberg & Federn, 1975, p. 276), titled "Contributions to a psychoanalytic exposition of melancholia." In this talk, Tausk anchored his reflections in two Freudian concepts that had profoundly influenced his thinking: first, the notion of mania as a substitute for affect; and second, the idea of libido detachment. These conceptual pillars framed his central inquiry, which revolved around two interrelated problems—namely, the dynamic relationship between melancholia and mania, and the theoretical understanding of melancholia as rooted in processes of libidinal withdrawal.

Regarding the first issue—the relationship between melancholia and mania—Tausk posited that the unconscious appears free to choose, at a certain point, between melancholic or manic expression. The content of the utterances remains essentially the same; what differs is their affective tone. Mood, he argued, is a function of libidinal cathexis—of both external objects and the subject's own person—and its manifestation depends on the developmental stage—narcissistic or autoerotic—from which this cathexis emerges during the illness.

To illustrate his points, Tausk presented two clinical cases. The first involved a female painter who experienced severe melancholia following the death of her father, and again 18 years later upon the loss of her sister. Notably, instead of progressing into a manic state, she exhibited signs of malice, spite, and aggression. According to Tausk, such manifestations were consistent across the anamneses of melancholic patients, which he characterized as fundamentally narcissistic. These patients often displayed grandiose self-regard cloaked in self-contempt. Genuine grandiose ideations—not merely reactive or compensatory ones—were also present, alongside a marked fear of excessive punishment, which suggested a latent sadomasochistic structure rooted in earlier infantile fantasies.

Tausk also addressed the relation between melancholia and *dementia praecox*. The nihilistic delusions common to melancholia—often somatically centered—he likened to the symbolic "organ speech" typical of schizophrenia. In melancholia, hallucinations frequently involve sensations related to the stomach, intestines, and smell. The patient's anxiety is not directed at the self as a unified whole, but specifically at the body, indicating a regressive fixation of the autoerotic libido on bodily organs. In contrast to schizophrenic patients, who attempt to adapt to this libidinal configuration through intellectual regression, melancholic patients retain intellectual integrity but are burdened by self-accusation. In melancholia, then, condemnation arises from a remnant of the narcissistic libidinal structure that resists such adaptation. This dynamic, according to Tausk, accounts for the melancholic's predilection for self-punishment, originating in the damming up of autoerotic libido. He further noted that the melancholic constitution is predominantly sadomasochistic and anally erotic.

Mania, in Tausk's view, is the inverse pole of melancholia. It embodies everything the melancholic accuses themselves of, but in an uninhibited, affectively unburdened form. In mania, judgment is suspended, giving way to unchecked behavior, aggression, and denial of any internal limitation. These individuals, being fundamentally autoerotic and narcissistic, often lack meaningful rapport with the analyst. Although they may have loved, Tausk argued, it was an unconscious attachment. Illness emerges at the moment these libidinal investments are relinquished, and without conscious awareness of this loss, personality structure fails to consolidate. In melancholia, the detached libido has not become sufficiently conscious to be reinvested. Tausk observed that older melancholic patients tend to fare worse than younger ones, attributing this to the latter's retained capacity for object love and psychic restitution.

Elaborating further, Rank invoked Karl Abraham (1877–1925), whose work proposed melancholia and mania as expressions of the same underlying complex. Rank also speculated whether the melancholic's bodily anxieties could be interpreted as a variant of death anxiety, albeit one that would require further theoretical clarification.

Nunberg revisited the issue—already touched upon by Tausk and Emil Kraepelin (1856–1926)—of whether one is dealing with melancholia as a primary condition or as it appears within broader psychopathological constellations. He suggested that the distinctive handwriting of melancholic patients may reflect incipient *dementia praecox*. Jekels and Hitschmann found the presentation lacking in its differentiation from certain hysterical syndromes. Jekels further questioned whether the melancholic's refusal to eat was necessarily due to feelings of unworthiness, and whether their anxiety was truly limited to the body alone.

Freud offered a nuanced response, noting that while some of Tausk's contributions were novel, others merely reiterated existing views. The defining feature of any disorder, Freud emphasized, lay not in the manifest symptoms—which rarely appear in isolation—but in their underlying mechanism. Observations of milder cases, as Hitschmann had indicated, offered the best chance of identifying the core structure of the illness. Freud reaffirmed that melancholia and mania are successive stages of the same condition. Melancholia represents a failed psychic attempt at adaptation; mania, by contrast, is a subsequent compensatory attempt. The melancholic's self-reproaches, he maintained, are originally directed at others and subsequently turned inward. Freud also cited a case of spontaneous remission to illustrate the crucial role of external precipitating factors. He likened the physiological correlate of melancholia to the affect of mourning, its necessary condition being the loss of a loved object. In melancholia, one cannot complete the work of mourning, perhaps because the love itself remains unconscious. Mania, as a reaction formation, declares the opposite: "I have not loved at all." Whether this repudiation is successful, Freud argued, hinges on the individual's ability to annihilate their superego. If the superego remains intact and continues to judge the ego against its previous state, melancholia persists.

Freud agreed that melancholia belonged among the narcissistic neuroses and acknowledged its resemblance to *dementia praecox* as a function of its libidinal structure. He further distinguished the anxiety of melancholia—what he termed "*organ anxiety*"—from other forms of anxiety. Narcissistic anxiety, Freud reminded the group of analysts gathered at the scientific meeting, stems from the castration complex, whereas melancholic anxiety manifests through somatic symptoms. Women suffering from melancholia, he noted, often appear anesthetic, reflecting a deflection of libido. He cautioned, however, that any coexisting organic pathology lay beyond the scope of psychoanalysis. Freud concluded by contrasting psychoses and neuroses: in the former, the entire libidinal apparatus is affected; in the latter, only the object-libido. Paranoia, he suggested, stands at the threshold, embodying a narcissistic struggle against object choice. Although disturbances in libido may appear secondary, he emphasized that no disorder of the ego can occur without a preceding disturbance in object relations. Hence, Freud affirmed, we are justified in regarding all ego disturbances as fundamentally libidinal in nature.

In his concluding remarks, Freud also acknowledged Tausk's earlier paper, "Compensation as a means of discounting the motive of repression" (Tausk, 1913c/1983a), recognizing it as one of the rare instances in which an economic perspective had been successfully integrated into the framework of psychoanalytic metapsychology (Freud, 1917/1979f).

Yet, as I have previously noted—and will now examine in greater depth—the outbreak of World War I marked a decisive rupture, redirecting both the personal aspirations and the clinical-professional trajectory of Viktor Tausk. What had until then been a period of vibrant intellectual exchange within the early psychoanalytic movement—marked by theoretical debates, creative tensions, and groundbreaking insights—was abruptly overshadowed by the imperatives of war, forcing many of its protagonists, Tausk among them, into radically altered roles and circumstances.

Service in World War I: Psychiatric Commitment to the Vulnerable (1915–1918)

In August 1915, shortly before being conscripted into military service, Tausk assembled a collection of his poems—previously published in various journals—with the intent of issuing them as a single volume. This project, however, ultimately remained unrealized. Earlier that spring, at Tausk's suggestion, his younger sister Nada had begun psychoanalytic treatment with Helene Deutsch due to difficulties in her romantic relationship. The analysis, however, ended abruptly after just a few weeks. Reportedly, Deutsch advised her to end the relationship, asserting that she was not genuinely in love—a claim that greatly upset Nada and led her to abandon the treatment altogether (Roazen, 1990, p. 77).

Between August 1915 and November 1918, during World War I, Tausk served first as chief psychiatrist and, from late 1916, as neurologist in Belgrade, then under Austro-Hungarian occupation. Despite the harsh wartime conditions, he remained intellectually active and deeply engaged with psychoanalytic inquiry. That same year, he published "On the psychology of the alcoholic occupation delirium" (Tausk, 1915/1983a; Roazen, 2017a), a paper that provoked lively debate within the Vienna Psychoanalytic Society (Nunberg & Federn, 1975, pp. 288–292). It is worth noting that in the fourth volume of the *Minutes*, the presentation appears under a slightly altered title—"On the psychology of alcoholic occupational delirium"—a variation that nevertheless refers to the same contribution.

In connection with his earlier-mentioned role as a military psychiatrist, Tausk once again turned to an in-depth exploration of melancholia. As discussed earlier, he had first presented on the topic before the Vienna Psychoanalytic Society on December 30, 1914. Two years later, at the beginning of 1916, drawing upon his clinical observations and reflections from the war front, he delivered a paper on January 19 at the Second Conference of

Medical Officers in Lublin, entitled “Diagnostische Erörterungen auf Grund der Zustandsbilder der sogenannten Kriegspsychosen” [Diagnostic considerations concerning the symptomatology of the so-called war psychoses] (Roazen, 2017a, pp. 119–140). In this presentation, Tausk advanced a nuanced understanding of melancholia as a pathological manifestation of narcissistic mechanisms underlying specific configurations of heterosexual-object choice.

Elaborating on Freud’s theory of narcissism, Tausk emphasized that while heterosexual libidinal investments may adopt a narcissistic structure, they do not lend themselves as readily to reabsorption into the ego in cases of object loss—unlike their homosexual counterparts, which may have originated in an exaggeratedly cathected ego. In melancholia, this asymmetry becomes clinically salient: the loss of the external love object is experienced as a collapse of self-love, leading to a profound disintegration of narcissistic structures—manifested in diminished self-esteem, depleted self-confidence, and affective destabilization.

With this theoretical foundation in place, Tausk introduced a number of diagnostic and conceptual insights that retain enduring relevance for psychoanalytically informed readers. He began by critically examining the term *war psychosis*, noting its initially indiscriminate diagnostic application by many clinicians. While some sought to isolate symptom constellations specific to wartime trauma, others employed the label with little theoretical precision. Over time, Tausk observed that what was frequently described as *war psychosis* was more accurately understood as the activation or exacerbation of pre-existing psychopathological structures—catalyzed, but not fundamentally transformed, by the traumatic circumstances of war.

According to Tausk’s extensive and multifaceted clinical experience, the diagnostic task was further complicated by sociolinguistic and cultural variables. The patients he encountered—drawn from the vast ethnic, linguistic, and socio-economic mosaic of the Austro-Hungarian monarchy—often presented with unfamiliar or ambiguous symptom formations. He emphasized the diagnostic challenges posed by limited language comprehension and by the cultural gulf separating urban-trained psychiatrists from rural conscripts. Many peasant patients, in particular, displayed rudimentary communicative capacities and impoverished symbolic repertoires, which rendered differential diagnosis—between, for instance, schizophrenia, mania, or general paresis—especially complex. Tausk underscored that behaviors such as fecal smearing or sudden violent outbursts might too hastily be interpreted as signs of schizophrenia in the absence of more elaborated symbolic expression.

Tausk’s observations reveal the profound variability in the clinical presentation of mental illness across social and cultural strata. He notes, for instance, that melancholia among his patients often appeared in a form of extreme inhibition—mute, somaticized, almost animal-like—devoid of introspective or symbolic content. Similarly, so-called functional disturbances such as neurasthenia, hysteria in its multiple forms, anxiety, and obsessional neurosis were not, as some contemporaries believed, confined to the educated classes. Rather, they also afflicted peasants and laborers alike. For Tausk, the determining factor was not intellectual sophistication but the vicissitudes of libidinal development. The recurrent emergence of mass hysteria across epochs and cultures revealed to him that such phenomena arise from archaic, foundational strata of the human psyche.

Building upon these clinical observations, Tausk turns to critique the prevailing classificatory models of psychiatry, which tended to isolate symptoms into rigid nosological entities—melancholia, paranoia, schizophrenia—while overlooking the fluid overlaps and mutual interpenetrations among them. In practice, he frequently encountered patients who defied such categorical clarity, displaying fully developed melancholic symptoms alongside elaborate paranoid delusions. These constellations did not simply juxtapose different disorders but intertwined them as co-dominant formations, casting doubt on the adequacy of fixed diagnostic frameworks.

Among Tausk's illustrative cases is that of a 34-year-old shoemaker from northern Bohemia who exhibited melancholic self-reproach, suicidal ideation, paranoid delusions of persecution, and pronounced hypochondriasis. Another striking example involved a noble officer whose life of manipulation and excess gave way to a melancholic state saturated with guilt and remorse—yet sustained a coherent paranoid structure of suspicion. In both cases, melancholia and paranoia emerged not as secondary traits but as autonomous, interacting psychopathologies. Such cases, Tausk insisted, demanded a subtler understanding of the psychodynamic mechanisms mediating their convergence or differentiation.

In this regard, Tausk's clinical orientation anticipates a more dynamic and structurally informed conception of psychosis—one that transcends descriptive symptomatology and probes the underlying psychic conflicts and developmental pathways shaping subjective experience. His diagnostic sensitivity foregrounds the influence of sociocultural, linguistic, and class variables while exposing the inherent limits of static nosological categories in capturing the lived complexity of mental suffering.

Indeed, Tausk's case material from the war front presents a diagnostic profile that destabilizes classical categorizations. His patients—manifesting syndromes ranging from melancholia and suicidal ideation to megalomania and persecutory delusions—often displayed affectively incompatible symptoms coexisting within the same psychic economy. Melancholic self-abasement, for instance, could paradoxically coexist with the grandiose delusions typical of paranoia. This tension—of simultaneous collapse and inflation—could not be explained through conscious content alone. Significantly, Tausk resists the impulse to propose a new category. Instead, he conceptualizes what he calls *paranoia cum melancholia* as a long-recognized but insufficiently theorized co-occurrence of two distinct libidinal pathologies, each governed by its own mechanism of withdrawal and defense.

As Freud had theorized in his seminal 1914 essay "On narcissism: An introduction," melancholia represents a pathological form of mourning. Following a suggestion by Ferenczi, Freud (1914b/1979e) noted that while both mourning and melancholia involve the withdrawal of libido from a lost object, only in melancholia is this libido redirected inward, toward the ego—a process of narcissistic reabsorption. The lost object is not relinquished but incorporated through identification, giving rise to self-reproaches that are, in truth, disguised attacks upon the internalized object.

Building upon this foundation, Tausk extends Freud's model by establishing a metapsychological bridge between melancholia and paranoia. Drawing on Freud's earlier analysis of the Schreber case (Freud, 1911/1980b), he reiterates that paranoia functions as a defense against unconscious homosexual impulses. The conditions of military life—intensely masculine, emotionally charged, and physically confined—amplify these latent currents. In such a milieu, libido is defensively withdrawn from homosexual cathexes to avert psychic disintegration, only to be redirected toward the ego, producing grandiosity, megalomania, and persecutory delusions. Projection thus becomes the dominant defense, externalizing intolerable internal conflict.

Melancholia, by contrast, follows an opposing libidinal trajectory. The self-reproaches characteristic of melancholia, though seemingly self-directed, are in fact veiled reproaches against the lost object. Through identification, the melancholic turns aggression inward, disguising hostility toward the beloved beneath the mask of self-condemnation. This mechanism accounts for the affective paralysis, masochistic resignation, and pervasive sense of worthlessness that define the melancholic condition.

From this comparative analysis, Tausk derives a striking hypothesis: paranoia and melancholia constitute two divergent responses to libidinal loss. The former processes homosexual-narcissistic cathexes through projection; the latter processes heterosexual-object cathexes through introjection. In *paranoia cum melancholia*, both currents coexist—the paranoid element transforming homosexual libido into persecutory ideation and inflated self-esteem, while the melancholic element converts heterosexual loss into self-directed despair.

Tausk's clinical findings consistently reinforce this dual model. In war neuroses, melancholic self-reproaches frequently revolved around female figures—mothers, wives, or lovers—whereas paranoid delusions arose primarily within homosocial contexts. He also noted that manic states often followed episodes of heterosexual frustration, serving as affective inversions that shielded the subject from melancholic collapse. The classical melancholic features—anhedonia, emotional blunting, and withdrawal from the natural world—thus appear as consequences of blocked heterosexual libidinal investment. When such libido cannot be reinvested, it becomes the substratum of depressive symptomatology, while libido withdrawn from homosexual cathexes is elaborated through paranoid defense.

In this theoretical horizon, Tausk (Roazen, 2017a, p. 132) recalls an unpublished hypothesis of Freud's—shared with him personally and with permission—which proves decisive for his metapsychological elaboration: individuals whose heterosexual-object choice is narcissistically structured may be particularly susceptible to melancholia. That is, when the heterosexual love object is not approached through libidinal differentiation but through narcissistic identification—analogous to the homosexual object—it becomes, upon loss, a direct threat to the integrity of the ego. The blow to narcissism, in such instances, acquires the devastating force of an injury rather than a mere bereavement. This hypothesis, Tausk observes, illuminates how melancholic and paranoid structures may emerge simultaneously within the same psychic economy.

Expanding upon Freud's suggestion, Tausk introduces a crucial refinement. Paranoia—traditionally regarded as the paradigmatic narcissistic-homosexual disorder—may also, he argues, reflect disturbances in narcissistically inflected heterosexual cathexes. Under extreme psychic strain, both libidinal configurations may collapse together. Such dual disintegration, often precipitated by the traumatic intensities of war, does not proceed gradually but rather as a sudden psychic implosion: the breakdown of homosexual investments pulling with it the destabilization of once-secure heterosexual positions. In this collapse, the apparent polarity between the two forms of libido reveals its illusory stability. Significantly, Tausk notes that many of his melancholic patients described enduring difficulties in establishing authentic heterosexual attachments, often traceable to early developmental fixations. These difficulties, he insists, should not be seen as consequences of melancholia but as predisposing libidinal vulnerabilities. The exacerbation of depressive states during sexual senescence—when the individual's capacity to function as love object or love subject wanes—further exposes the narcissistic fragility underpinning these investments. Tausk even observes that some melancholic women exhibit the emergence of secondary masculine traits during depressive episodes, which he interprets as somatic expressions of libidinal reconfiguration and potential shifts toward homosexual identification.

While acknowledging that paranoia and melancholia may, in some instances, appear in isolation, Tausk speculates that "pure" clinical forms are often deceptive, masking deeper and more entangled libidinal histories. In slowly progressing paranoia, he proposes, the gradual erosion of heterosexual investments leaves too little libido to sustain melancholic identification. Conversely, in the sudden psychic shocks of wartime neuroses, the collapse of one libidinal system can instantaneously precipitate the collapse of the other: homosexual disintegration triggering heterosexual implosion, and vice versa.

To ground this theoretical architecture in clinical observation, Tausk introduces the notion of *acute anxiety paranoia*—a war-specific psychosis characterized by persecutory ideation, intense anxiety, and profound social withdrawal, particularly prevalent among soldiers drawn from culturally or linguistically marginalized populations. Such syndromes, he argues, often remit with a change of environment, suggesting that they function as defensive responses to the intolerable psychological demands of military existence. Within this dynamic, paranoia operates as a protective screen against repressed homosexual-narcissistic threats, transforming unbearable internal tension into persecutory representations projected onto the external world.

In conclusion, Tausk directs a sharp critique toward the prevailing methods of descriptive psychiatry. Devoid of psychoanalytic understanding—of unconscious wishes, infantile defenses, and the complex vicissitudes of libido—traditional nosology, he argues, remains ill-equipped to comprehend these intricate clinical realities. The cases he presents refuse to fit neatly within conventional categories, oscillating instead between melancholia, paranoia, hysteria, and obsessional neurosis. For Tausk, the way forward does not lie in multiplying diagnostic labels but in returning to psychoanalytic inquiry itself. Only through such a lens can these syndromes be apprehended not as static pathologies but as dynamic outcomes of libidinal conflict, defense, and the ever-shifting equilibria of the ego.

While his theoretical contributions reached a moment of particular clarity, Tausk's personal circumstances took a more somber turn. On March 23, 1916, his father, Hermann Tausk, died. Around the same time, the passing of the father of Martha—Viktor's former wife—left her in severe financial difficulty. Amid the wartime privations, she was compelled to seek employment, a formidable task under such conditions. Martha, an active member of the Social Democratic Party since 1911, would later become a prominent figure in the Austrian Parliament's Upper Chamber (Eissler, 1983, p. 26), but at that time she faced grave distress. Their children were placed temporarily in a care facility in Bohemia. In an effort to mitigate the family's suffering, Viktor's mother, Emilie, encouraged Martha to relocate to Zagreb, where food supplies were reportedly more accessible.

Tausk continued to correspond with Martha from the front. In a letter dated September 30, he lamented his inability to visit her due to financial constraints and confessed to being emotionally depleted, with little strength remaining to maintain his psychological balance. He expressed uncertainty about the internal resources he might draw upon to rebuild his life—once again—after the war (Roazen, 1990). By late November, he was stationed in Lublin, Poland—then under Austro-Hungarian control—continuing his work as a military psychiatrist. Despite profound emotional and financial hardship, Tausk persevered, sustained in part by his continued engagement with writing and private clinical work outside his official duties.

It was during this period that Edoardo Weiss encountered Tausk again. Weiss, then overseeing a hospital train transporting wounded soldiers from the Russian front to Lublin, was approached by Tausk after the patients had disembarked. Recalling the encounter, Weiss (1991, p. 11) described his friend as profoundly depressed and pessimistic about the outcome of the war. Tausk predicted the irreversible defeat of the Central Powers and envisioned Vienna as the fading capital of a collapsing empire—one in which psychoanalysts would find little opportunity to earn a living. He also confided a more intimate grief: his fiancée's betrayal through infidelity, a wound made all the more painful given the seriousness of their engagement.

Years later, when he learned of Tausk's tragic death, Weiss admitted that although he was shaken and saddened, he was not surprised (Weiss, 1991, p. 11). In a letter to Roazen dated July 1, 1966, Weiss remarked that Tausk believed Freud did not want him to live—a belief Weiss attributed to what he considered the darker side of Freud's personality (Roazen, 1977). Four years later, Weiss further clarified that Tausk likely felt abandoned by those closest to him, particularly Freud (Weiss, 1991, p. 11).

Yet, even amid such turmoil, Tausk exhibited extraordinary moral courage. One notable instance involved Fritz Weiss, a young soldier sentenced to death for refusing to participate in the execution of enemy prisoners. Tausk intervened, arguing that Fritz had acted on moral principle and that punishing him was a profound injustice. Many years later, in South America, Tausk's youngest son, Victor Hugo, met Fritz again. Deeply moved, Fritz still kept a photograph of Tausk displayed in his home, in gratitude for the act that had once saved his life (Roazen, 1990, p. 61).

Tausk's experience with such cases informed his essay "On the psychology of the war deserter" (Tausk, 1916c/1983a), which he later presented as a lecture on March 3, 1917, in Belgrade during the Ninth Military Medicine Evening. That year, Tausk also published "On a particular form of obsessive fantasies" (Tausk, 1916a/1983a), a piece included in the Spanish edition that compiles his psychoanalytic writings (Tausk, 1983a), though notably absent from the corresponding English edition. In addition to this article, he authored "Contributions to the psychopathology of everyday life" (Tausk, 1916b/1983a) and "Some comments on Abraham's paper on 'ejaculatio praecox'" (Tausk, 1917/1983a). In his correspondence with Freud, Abraham expressed appreciation for Tausk's insights on the latter essay, while simultaneously criticizing "On the psychology of the war deserter" (Tausk, 1916c/1983a) for its verbosity and lack of conceptual precision (Freud & Abraham, 1965/1979).

In late 1916, Tausk was transferred back to Belgrade, an active military zone. There, he formed a warm relationship with Kosa Lazarević, a young Serbian widow. Using his military rank, Tausk secured her release after she was detained by soldiers for allegedly insulting the Austrian army. In gratitude—and owing to her family's prominence—she offered to help him secure a professorship in psychiatry, either in Belgrade or Zagreb. Though initially leaning toward Belgrade, where he felt greater cultural affinity with the Serbs than the Croats, Tausk ultimately declined to marry her, just as he had done previously with Lea Rosen in Berlin—despite the fact that such a union might have stabilized his personal and financial circumstances (Roazen, 1990).

During Christmas 1916, Tausk's son, Marius, was sent to live with a family in Graz, Austria, where he would remain until completing his medical studies in 1926. Two years later, his mother and younger brother, Victor Hugo, also moved to Graz. Sadly, Victor Hugo would later pass away there (M. Tausk, 1973). Although Marius initially aspired to follow in his father's footsteps as a psychiatrist, he later abandoned this ambition, unable to overcome the trauma of his father's suicide. Early in 1917, the family faced further adversity: both children were expelled from school, in part due to Marius's outspoken views on religion and Victor Hugo's mischief. Nevertheless, by mid-1918, the relatively optimistic atmosphere within the Austrian military regarding their position in Serbia allowed officers to bring their families. That summer, Tausk's children rejoined him in Belgrade (Roazen, 1990).

Throughout this period, Tausk made repeated trips to Vienna in order to maintain his connection with the Vienna Psychoanalytic Society. On January 6, 1918, he presented to the Society what would become his most significant and enduring contribution: "On the origin of the 'influencing machine' in schizophrenia" (Tausk, 1919/1983a). Curiously, this presentation is not recorded in the *Minutes* of the Society. The last documented contribution by Tausk in that record remains his presentation of March 31, 1915, previously mentioned, titled "On the psychology of alcoholic occupational delirium" (Nunberg & Federn, 1975, p. xiii).

Regardless of this editorial omission, the paper on the "influencing machine" was extensively discussed by the Society two weeks after its delivery and was published the following year. In this landmark essay, Tausk sought to illuminate the structure and genesis of schizophrenic delusions through the lens of psychoanalytic theory—at a time when such conceptual tools were still fragmented and lacked systematic articulation. His formulation anticipated and ultimately contributed to the development of Freud's second topographical model of the mind (Birman, 1990).

After the war, Tausk remained in Belgrade for a short time before relocating to Budapest, where he presented his paper "Psychoanalysis and the capacity for judgment" at the Fifth International Psychoanalytic Congress, convened on September 28 and 29, 1918. During the congress, it became evident that he was suffering from serious psychological distress—a state Freud later acknowledged in his obituary, citing Tausk's marked irritability and suggesting a dysthymic episode. One of the key proposals debated at the congress was the requirement that all practicing analysts undergo personal analysis. Introduced by Herman Nunberg, the motion was rejected at the time, largely due to opposition from Tausk and Rank. Seven years later, however, at the Ninth IPA Congress, which met in Bad Homburg between September 2 and 5, 1925, the proposal was finally adopted as a formal requirement. This requirement remains paradoxical, given that several founding figures of the movement, including Freud himself, as well as Federn, Rank, and Ferenczi, had not undergone full analyses (Sánchez-Barranco,

1996). Also raised at the congress was the question of whether psychoanalysts needed to be medically trained—a position strongly favored by the American delegation. Whereas the American psychoanalytic movement pursued integration within medical institutions, the European contingent remained more open to non-medical practitioners. Freud, for his part, consistently worked to differentiate psychoanalysis from the field of medicine—possibly to protect the clinical work of his daughter and close collaborators, or perhaps as a reaction to his own alienation from the academic medical establishment.

Freud emphasized the vital importance of self-analysis as a preparatory step for future analysts. He articulated this view in "The future prospects of psychoanalytic therapy" (Freud, 1910/1979c) and "Recommendations to physicians practicing psychoanalysis" (Freud, 1912b/1980d). Later, in *Analysis Terminable and Interminable* (Freud, 1937/1980g), Freud went further, proposing that analysts should, without hesitation or stigma, undergo periodic re-analyses—perhaps every five years—to ensure continued clarity and insight in their work.

Decades later, Janet Malcolm (1981), in *Psychoanalysis: The Impossible Profession*, revisited many of the enduring questions surrounding psychoanalytic technique. Through a series of interviews with practicing analysts, she illuminated the intricacies of clinical work, offering not only a lucid reflection on the inherent challenges of the profession but also a bold exercise in self-critique from within the analytic community.

Returning to Tausk's biography: the day after the armistice was signed in Padua, Italy—marking the end of World War I on November 3, 1918—he returned to Vienna and began the difficult task of rebuilding his life. According to Roazen (1971/1978a), he may have considered applying for the title of *Privatdozent*, an academic designation allowing one to lecture independently at the university level. However, no formal record of such an application exists in the archives of the University of Vienna (Eissler, 1983). In any case, Tausk resumed his psychiatric practice. As previously mentioned, he had the option of continuing his work in Yugoslavia, where he had even been offered a professorship. Yet accepting that post would have entailed severing his ties with Freud and the Vienna psychoanalytic circle—an outcome he clearly sought to avoid. Remaining in Vienna, however, came at significant personal and financial cost. Once again, he fell into a profound depression, no doubt exacerbated by his persistent economic difficulties.

On December 7, 1918, Freud referred a patient to Tausk—although this patient was unable to pay for treatment. Nevertheless, not long thereafter, Tausk was reportedly seeing seven patients a day, six of whom could afford to pay for their sessions. Despite the burdens he bore, he continued to pursue his analytic work with determination and resilience.

Freud's Refusal to Analyze Tausk, Helene Deutsch's Failed Analysis, and Suicide as Expiation (1919)

I now arrive at the final year of Viktor Tausk's life—a year overshadowed by mounting personal turmoil and culminating in his suicide. In the months leading up to this tragic end, Tausk sent six letters to Freud, dated January 22 and 29, March 1 and 30, April 12, and May 31. While these letters illuminate, with striking clarity, the deepening complexity of Tausk's inner world, Eissler (1983) maintains that they reveal no explicit conflict or overt tension in his correspondence with Freud during this period. Nevertheless, these months were marked by two painful rejections that weighed heavily on Tausk: Freud's refusal to accept him as an analytic patient and his denial of Tausk's request for the treatment of his son, Marius. Although, according to Roazen (1990), Tausk's formal request for analysis was made in 1918, a letter from Ferenczi to Freud dated August 24, 1914, indicates that Freud had already declined this possibility several years earlier:

> I promise to muster everything, in order to mitigate the difficulties on account of which you decline to analyze Tausk. If things turn out differently to some extent, then that would be material for further analysis, whereby you would have to proceed with all necessary strictness.
>
> (Falzeder et al., 1996, p. 15)

Despite Tausk's renewed petition, Freud remained resolute in his refusal. Instead, he advised that Tausk enter analysis with either Paul Federn or Eduard Hitschmann—recommendations that Tausk ultimately declined. Freud further proposed Helene Deutsch as an alternative (Eissler, 1971; Hamilton, 1991), although Roazen (1990) contends that this suggestion may, in fact, have originated with Freud himself. The motives underlying Freud's steadfast refusal to undertake Tausk's analysis remain intricate and continue to elicit considerable scholarly discussion. What can be established with some certainty, however, is Freud's unmistakable personal antipathy toward Tausk—a sentiment that exceeded mere theoretical disagreement. This aversion finds vivid corroboration in the undated reminiscences of Ludwig Jekels, himself a psychoanalyst, Freud's analysand, and a close Polish colleague of Helene Deutsch.

These recollections (Jekels, n.d.), preserved in the Siegfried Bernfeld Papers (Container 17, Library of Congress), appear to have been written in response to Bernfeld's inquiries while preparing the Freud biography he ultimately never completed. In *Early psychoanalytic reminiscences*, Jekels provides unique insights into the personal and institutional tensions within the early Viennese analytic community, documenting Freud's explicit refusal to analyze Tausk and capturing the subtle dynamics among Freud's closest collaborators.

In these typed reminiscences (p. 8), Jekels recounts that when he directly asked Freud why he refused to take Tausk into analysis, Freud answered bluntly: "*He is going to kill me!*" (Gay, 1988, p. 703). Freud's deep mistrust of Tausk also surfaces in letters to Fritz Wittels and Paul Federn, where he described Tausk metaphorically as "a chained dog."

Further insights into this fraught relationship are offered by Roazen (1992, p. 173), who explains that Jekels—like Tausk himself—resented the changing dynamics within Freud's circle following the internationalization of psychoanalysis. According to Jekels, tensions intensified after 1910, when the meetings of the Vienna Psychoanalytic Society were relocated from Freud's private apartment—where, as he recalls, "the atmosphere was on the whole a rather agreeable, instructive one and full of enjoyment"—to the hall of the Vienna College of Physicians. Jekels describes the shift in terms that highlight growing rivalries and personal antagonisms:

> Unfortunately, this changed markedly when the sessions were transferred into the hall of the Vienna College of Physicians. There differences came to the fore which to my mind had various personal motives as their basis; above all, there was one to be the favorite son [of Freud] and to cut out others who were in favor with him. Sad to say, in this attempt the usual parliamentary forms were often greatly transgressed. Most often this happened between Stekel and Sadger; later Tausk also entered the lists, who loved to assail the two of them. This went so far that Freud asked me after one of the sessions: "What does Tausk want from Sadger; he is indeed a serious scholar!" Besides, Freud thought very highly of Tausk's analytical talents yet refused firmly to analyze him although Tausk had asked him repeatedly to do it; I too asked Freud to do that, but he replied: "He is going to kill me."
>
> (Jekels, n.d., as cited in Roazen, 1992, p. 173)

Building upon these archival insights, Roazen (1971/1978a, 1990) further supports the view—drawing on interviews with Paul Federn, Helene Deutsch, Richard Sterba (1898–1989), and Philip Sarasin (1888–1968)—that Freud regarded Tausk as psychologically dangerous, fearing he might co-opt Freud's intellectual contributions. Deutsch later corroborated this impression, recalling that Freud believed Tausk possessed an exceptional ability to absorb the ideas of others and subsequently present them as his own, sometimes even accusing colleagues of plagiarism when similar ideas resurfaced. This dispute over intellectual authorship was not new. As early as 1913, Tausk confided to Edoardo Weiss his conviction that Freud undervalued his originality and had appropriated certain conceptual insights. Weiss, however, found Tausk's complaint ironic, recalling an earlier episode in which Tausk had done something strikingly similar to him. Tausk even hesitated to share particular insights with Freud, fearing that they might be misused or absorbed without acknowledgment. In the 1930s, Weiss himself experienced what he perceived as Freud's "selective memory," when Freud failed to credit him in one of his publications. By 1965, Weiss relayed this memory to Roazen, though he was no longer able to recall the specific details. To clarify the incident, Weiss sent a follow-up letter on October 20, 1969—a letter Roazen would later generously share with me.

In that letter, Weiss wrote to Roazen:

> "Many colleagues ask me about the plagiarism you mention in a footnote. I cannot remember what I told you about it. I would be very grateful to you if you could remind me of what I told you."
>
> (E. Weiss, personal communication, October 20, 1969)

Roazen's own reply remains undisclosed, as he shared only Weiss's letter with me, not his correspondence. As Roazen revealed in a letter dated May 22, 1997:

> "I am afraid I do not usually keep copies of my own letters; presumably that letter in response to Weiss is in his papers, now open at the Library of Congress in Washington."
>
> (P. Roazen, personal communication, May 22, 1997)

Despite this lead—and follow-up inquiries with Weiss's sons, Emilio and Guido—I was unable to locate Roazen's reply. In his personal communication to me, Emilio conveyed information gathered from both himself and his brother, noting that most of their father's documents are archived at the US National Academy of Sciences (E. Weiss, personal communication, June 18, 1997). Roazen (1982) notes that although he had full access to Weiss's interviews with Eissler, those materials remain embargoed until 2057 and are housed at the Library of Congress. Eissler (1974) later accessed both letters and judged Roazen's response insufficient to resolve the matter. However, nine years afterward, Eissler (1983) identified the relevant work as "A disturbance of memory on the Acropolis" (Freud, 1936/1979j), where Freud addressed derealization as a defense mechanism—an idea Weiss had earlier introduced. Weiss later elaborated on the theme in *Agoraphobia in the Light of Ego Psychology* (Weiss, 1964), though his preliminary thoughts appeared in "Regression and projection in the superego" (Weiss, 1932), possibly unaware that Freud had touched on related phenomena in "Fetishism" (Freud, 1927/1979i).

Regarding Tausk's emotional response to Freud's refusal to analyze him, the available evidence remains indirect. According to his son, Victor Hugo, the refusal inflicted a profound insult and narcissistic wound—an interpretation he received either from Jelka or from Eduard Hitschmann, his own analyst and a close friend of his father. Years later, this account was relayed to Paul Roazen, who, accompanied by his wife, visited the Netherlands and interviewed both Victor Hugo and Tausk's sister Nada. In a subsequent conversation, Helene Deutsch confirmed that Freud's rejection had left an enduring scar, describing Tausk as deeply humiliated (Roazen, 1977).

Nevertheless, in January 1919, Tausk agreed to enter analysis with Helene Deutsch, becoming her first analytic patient (Hamilton, 1991). This was remarkable, considering that, while Deutsch possessed substantial psychiatric experience from seven years at the Wagner-Jauregg Clinic, she was still a newcomer to psychoanalysis. Her position at the clinic had already been exceptional, as women were typically barred from such posts. Roazen (1990) notes that upon her departure, Wagner-Jauregg issued a certificate—dated November 12, 1918—referring to her as an "almost assistant," a formulation designed to circumvent existing legal restrictions.

At that time, Deutsch had already begun her own analysis with Freud, three months before taking on Tausk as a patient, succeeding Dr. Erzsébet Radó-Révész (1887–1923)—a Hungarian neurologist and psychoanalyst, and the wife of Sándor Radó (1890–1972), the Hungarian analyst whom Freud initially favored but later regarded with displeasure (Roazen & Swerdloff, 1977). This circumstance created a uniquely intricate configuration: Freud analyzed Deutsch, who in turn analyzed Tausk. According to Roazen (1990), a tacit understanding underpinned this arrangement, allowing Freud to maintain indirect influence. Deutsch herself would later describe the situation as a "diabolical agreement" (Roazen, 1978b).

Tausk's analysis with Deutsch proceeded with remarkable intensity—six sessions per week, with fees paid in accordance with psychoanalytic convention (Roazen, 1992). By March 1919, barely three months after it had begun, Freud intervened, arguing that Tausk's frequent references to him made it impossible for Deutsch to continue the treatment. At Freud's insistence, Deutsch reluctantly terminated Tausk's analysis (Bentinck van Schoonheten, 2013/2016, p. 235).

Shortly thereafter, Freud also decided that Deutsch should discontinue her own analysis with him. When she expressed her wish to continue, Freud referred her to Ferenczi. She declined this recommendation because relocating to Budapest would have created serious linguistic difficulties for her son, Martin. Freud then suggested Hanns Sachs, but she rejected this option as well. She ultimately entered analysis with Karl Abraham (Roazen, 1971/1978a).

Freud's relationship with Deutsch also suffered when her husband, Felix Deutsch, concealed the severity of Freud's palatal cancer—a breach that extended tensions beyond the clinic.

In March 1919, Viktor Tausk suffered yet another disappointment when Freud refused to take his eldest son, Marius, into analysis, fearing it might hinder the boy's natural development. In a letter dated April 12, Tausk acknowledged Freud's decision, noting that Marius himself had declined the offer. Enclosed with his father's correspondence, Marius's brief note affirmed his own independence and requested that the letter be returned to his father at the following Wednesday meeting (Eissler, 1983). Earlier, on March 30, Tausk had reported Marius was struggling with obsessive thoughts and distressing nightmares. Kanzer (1971), however, argued Marius's condition was general and likely compounded by alcohol, although Marius—an active member of an anti-alcohol league—denied use.

Compounding his emotional turmoil was a series of romantic disappointments, often involving Jewish women such as Luci von Jacobi, Else Jerusalem, and Sonja Drublowicz. His inability to commit fueled depressive episodes. In an interview with Heinz Winnik, Lea Rosen recalled Tausk admitted to enjoying humiliating a romantic partner and having a disturbing preference for young, virginal women (Eissler, 1974, 1983).

In the months preceding his suicide on July 3, 1919, Tausk began a relationship with Hilde Loewi (1895–1976), 16 years his junior, a former patient and concert pianist. According to Eissler (1974), she became pregnant, and Tausk planned to marry her to avoid scandal. Following his death and several failed abortion attempts, the termination ultimately occurred (Roazen, 1972).

This account is corroborated by a letter Olga Knopf (1889–1978) sent to Anna Freud on June 12, 1970. In it, Knopf recalled that, in the spring of 1919, Viktor Tausk brought a young woman to her office, introducing her as his sister-in-law. Upon examination, Knopf confirmed the woman's pregnancy and performed an emergency abortion, which ultimately failed. She later visited the patient—whom she subsequently identified as Hilde—on two occasions at Tausk's office, noting her evident fear and profound sadness.

Shortly thereafter, Tausk confided his intention to marry Hilde, thereby revealing the earlier deception. About two months later, Hilde was admitted to the pathological pregnancy ward of the Women's Clinic at the University of Vienna's General Hospital, then directed by Friedrich Schauta (1849–1919), with Ludwig Adler (1876–1958) serving as acting head. It was Adler who arranged her transfer into Knopf's care. At that time, Hilde was four months pregnant and had developed a uterine wall tumor requiring a vaginal cesarean section. She recovered well following the operation. During her hospitalization, Hilde reportedly confided to Knopf that she had been seduced by Tausk during her very first analytic session, and that she had been a virgin prior to the encounter. This painful disclosure was later corroborated by Thérèse Neyant-Sutterman in an interview with Marius Tausk, conducted in Nijmegen (the Netherlands) in December 1978 (Neyant-Sutterman, 1978).

Fifteen years later, in 1934, Hilde married and subsequently left Vienna; although the union remained childless, those who knew the couple described it as harmonious. She died of ovarian cancer in 1976. Her husband later supplied Eissler with additional biographical detail, including personal descriptions of her appearance (Eissler, 1983).

The sequence of events suggests that Tausk's engagement to Hilde failed to bring him the emotional equilibrium he so desperately sought. This is poignantly reflected in Roazen's (1990) historical reconstruction of his final hours. On July 2, 1919—the day before his suicide—Tausk wrote to Freud excusing himself from the Wednesday meeting of the Vienna Psychoanalytic Society. He explained that he had pressing personal matters to address and wished to resolve them independently, without turning to Freud for guidance. That same afternoon, Tausk spent time with his eldest son, Marius, who had traveled from Graz. During their conversation, he advised Marius not to live according to rigid ideals or prescribed patterns—a remark possibly directed at his former wife, Martha. Notably, despite any bitterness she may have harbored, Martha never spoke ill of Viktor to their children and remained committed to preserving a positive image of their father (Eissler, 1983). Later that day, Tausk also wrote to his sister Nada, then in Yugoslavia, thanking her for the cigarettes and bacon she had sent. He mentioned his forthcoming marriage—a chilling irony, given that he would end his life just hours later.

According to Marius—albeit with some uncertainty—Tausk may have attended a concert that evening with Hilde. Outwardly, nothing in their activities seemed to foreshadow the impending tragedy. Yet what passed between Tausk and Hilde that night remains unknown. Given Tausk's psychological instability, a quarrel cannot be ruled out. On the morning of July 3, 1919, Viktor Tausk ended his life by simultaneously hanging and shooting himself. He left behind a will and two letters—one addressed to Freud, the other to Hilde. Upon receiving news, Ilka (also known as Jelka) was informed, and she had her husband send a telegram to Martha in Graz, stating that her former husband was gravely ill. A second telegram, conveying news of his death, followed hours later—but by then, Martha had already departed for Vienna with her children (Roazen, 1990).

Two days later, on July 5, Marius called at Freud's home, seeking some understanding of his father's death. Freud received him briefly, between appointments. In that restrained and somewhat distant encounter, he mentioned that he had received a letter from Viktor Tausk shortly before the suicide and would forward it in due time. On a subsequent visit, Anna Freud delivered both the farewell letter and the complete correspondence between Freud and his father. As Roazen (1990) later noted, Freud seemed eager to close this chapter, as though returning the papers might seal the emotional and intellectual bond that had long unsettled him.

Tausk, by contrast, felt no apparent compulsion to erase or repudiate the traces of his relationship with Freud. His final letter—dated July 3, 1919—reveals instead a remarkable composure, a serenity that borders on transcendence. It speaks of gratitude rather than reproach, of care for others rather than self-pity. In this letter, Tausk entrusts Freud with a paternal role, asking him to look after Hilde and his children, while extending warm wishes to the Psychoanalytic Society and to all who had once helped him. It is as though, in the shadow of death, he sought reconciliation not only with Freud but with the analytic world that had both inspired and excluded him. As Roazen (1990, pp. 127–128) records, Tausk wrote:

> Please render assistance to my beloved fiancée, Miss Hilde Loewi (11 Körnergasse 2), the dearest woman who ever entered into my life. She

> will not ask much of you, because she has a great capacity for happiness within herself, but she tends toward compulsive symptoms and identifications. She is noble, pure, and kind; it is worth the trouble to give her good advice.
>
> I thank you for all the good which you have done me. It was much and had given meaning to the last ten years of my life. Your work is genuine and great, I shall take leave of this life knowing that I was one of those who witnessed the triumph of one of the greatest ideas of mankind.
>
> I have no melancholy, my suicide is the healthiest, most decent deed of my unsuccessful life. I have no accusations against anyone, my heart is without resentment, I am only dying somewhat earlier than I would have died naturally.
>
> I greet the Psychoanalytic Association, I wish it well with all my heart. I thank all those who helped me when I was in need. Those who have claim to this gratitude will know it for themselves.
>
> I hope you will have a long life, in health, strong and capable of working […] Please, also look after my sons from time to time.

The tone of this letter is both moving and enigmatic. Its apparent calm suggests a man who, facing psychic dissolution, strives to impose meaning upon chaos—transforming despair into dignity. Yet beneath the serenity lies the muted echo of unbearable psychic conflict: the tension between gratitude and exclusion, between identification with the father and the wish to break free from his symbolic authority. Although the letter conveys no explicit account of the intrapsychic mechanisms leading to his suicide, such dynamics emerge more clearly in Tausk's testament, where he confesses his inability to protect either himself or Hilde from harm, and the intolerable fatigue of sustaining a persona that exceeded his emotional and psychological resources. For his eldest son, Marius Tausk, these reasons alone sufficed to explain his father's death. In later reflections, he sought to temper the posthumous controversy surrounding Freud's role, remarking that the issue had seemed of little significance until Paul Roazen's *Brother Animal* (Roazen, 1969) first drew public attention to it.

In his will, Viktor Tausk requested that all his writings be destroyed—a wish his younger son, Victor Hugo, dutifully fulfilled over the course of an entire day. He appointed Camillo Gans as executor of his estate and designated Eduard Hitschmann—an internist and early member of the Vienna Psychoanalytic Society—as guardian of his sons. This decision was far from incidental: as previously noted, Hitschmann was not only Victor Hugo's analyst but also one of Tausk's closest personal friends, making him a natural and deeply trusted choice to oversee the children's welfare. Among his final directives, Tausk urged Hitschmann to ensure that both boys receive psychoanalytic treatment, convinced they displayed early signs of neurotic vulnerability. True to this wish, Hitschmann provided Victor

Hugo with free psychoanalytic treatment from September 1923 to February 1924 (Roazen, 1990).

That same day, news of Tausk's death reached Paul Federn, who—profoundly shaken—wrote a personal letter to his wife, Wilma Federn (1884–1949, née Bauer), then convalescing in the countryside. Despite their past rivalries—rooted partly in their shared desire for Freud's recognition (Eissler, 1974) and perhaps complicated by Tausk's flirtations with the much younger Wilma—Federn's reaction was one of genuine grief and affection. The emotional candor of his letter testifies to the intricate web of admiration, competition, and latent tenderness that long defined his relationship with Tausk, a dynamic emblematic of Freud's inner circle, where loyalty and envy so often intertwined.

Decades later, in early October 2000, Ernst Federn, son of Paul Federn, would confirm this enduring bond in a letter to me, writing:

> "Tausk and Federn were intimate friends. Tausk flirted with Federn's wife, which led to difficulties, but Freud intervened, and Tausk and Federn remained friends."
>
> (E. Federn, personal communication, October 3, 2000)

This enduring regard for Tausk, coupled with Paul Federn's capacity to question Freud's idealized image, imbues the letter he wrote on the very day of Tausk's death with striking moral and emotional clarity. Addressed to Wilma, then convalescing in the countryside, the letter reads in part:

> I must write you the worst. Today Tausk shot himself. I don't yet know anything more detailed [...] I am so terribly sorry about him. If I had been able, I would certainly have helped him, although he always bit the hand that reached out to help him. I had forgiven him inwardly, but I was no longer fond of him after the time he so insulted me, and at every opportunity—even after Budapest—whenever I approached him in a friendly way I found only vanity, envy, and lack of interest. If Freud had shown him a human interest, not simply recognition and support, he might have continued his martyr-like existence [...] But he was not kind, as little as Freud is kind, i.e., Freud possesses so much love for people that he can be kind, but in his old age he became increasingly harder—and this is understandable with Freud because he, too, had to live a life unworthy of his greatness—That we could not keep Tausk is our shame. However, he made enemies for himself everywhere and always; at the end he drove his psychological patients away, apparently in order to demonstrate the uselessness of the method, out of rancour against Freud.
>
> (P. Federn, 1919, letter to his wife Wilma, as cited in Roazen, 1990, p. 153).

The letter was later made available to Paul Roazen by Ernst Federn, under the express condition that it be reproduced only in part. The excerpts published here comprise those passages directly concerning Tausk, authorized for limited circulation. Yet Roazen ultimately declined to adhere to that agreement, asserting that scholarly integrity demanded full transparency rather than selective omission. This decision, however, provoked Ernst Federn's disapproval (Federn, 1973), who argued that compliance with the original understanding might not only have safeguarded his father's posthumous reputation but also spared Tausk's children the renewed anguish of revisiting such painful memories. Ernst's concern found an unexpected echo in Anna Freud's position. She, too, chose to withhold certain materials pertaining to her father's views on Tausk, seeking to protect the coherence—and perhaps the moral dignity—of Freud's legacy (Roazen, 1990).

Five days after his initial letter, Federn mentioned Tausk once more in a letter to his wife. In this second correspondence, he confided that he was currently treating one of Tausk's former patients and expressed deep discomfort at the prospect of visiting the bereaved family. He admitted to lacking the emotional strength to speak to them with sincerity. Nonetheless, seven years later, in 1926, when Marius Tausk was invited to attend a meeting of the Vienna Psychoanalytic Society, he was received with warmth and kindness by Federn—who, years afterward, in 1950, would himself die by suicide with a gunshot to the head (Roazen, 1990).

Tausk was buried the day after his death, without religious rites, in Vienna's Central Cemetery. The solemnity of the event was disrupted by an emotional outburst from Camillo Gans, who, visibly distressed, could not comprehend why Martha had allowed Hilde to lead the funeral procession alongside her. He interpreted this gesture as a sign of disrespect toward Viktor. That same day, the *Neue Wiener Journal*—a newspaper to which Tausk had previously contributed—published an obituary that paid respectful tribute to his life and work (Eissler, 1983).

Freud's reaction to Tausk's suicide remains enveloped in ambiguity, shaped by striking inconsistencies between his public pronouncements and private communications. Read together, these disparate sources offer only a partial, yet nonetheless valuable, glimpse into the complex and often conflicted sentiments he harbored toward his former disciple. In this regard, Eissler (1971) offered a perceptive hypothesis:

> I would surmise that the discrepancy between the objective portrait of Tausk that Freud, in his role as quasi-historian, left to posterity and the subjective one that he had formed out of his personal contacts with the deceased was one of the reasons why Tausk's obituary was published over the signature of "editor's office" (*Die Redaktion*).
>
> (p. 104)

Eissler (1971) further observed—in a revealing footnote—that Roazen believed Freud adopted this strategy to diffuse personal responsibility for Tausk's suicide. Supporting this interpretation, Eissler meticulously cataloged Freud's authorship of obituaries: of the eight Freud composed (including Tausk's), seven appeared in the *Internationale Zeitschrift für Psychoanalyse.* Among these, one was signed by "the editor," another by "the editorial office and editor," one by "the editor Freud," another by "Freud," and two by "Sigm. Freud" (p. 104).

Within Freud's public record, the most consequential of these remarks is the obituary for Tausk that appeared in the *Internationale Zeitschrift für Psychoanalyse*, attributed at the time to *Die Redaktion* (The Editorial Committee). However, James Strachey (1887–1967)—editor of *The Standard Edition of the Complete Psychological Works of Sigmund Freud* later identified Freud as its true author. He confirmed this attribution in a personal letter to Paul Roazen, dated January 28, 1967, the very year of his own death. I was able to examine the content of this letter thanks to Roazen's generosity in sharing a copy with me. While Roazen (1990) acknowledged the letter's existence (p. 134), he chose not to reproduce it in full.

What follows is the complete transcription of that letter—presented here for the first time—allowing the reader to weigh its historical and psychoanalytic significance without mediation:

> Dear Dr. Roazen,
>
> I am very sorry that, as you guess, your letter was overlooked in the general confusion that accompanied our return from the West Indies last spring. In any case, however, I had (and have) no information to give you.
>
> I have no reason in particular for attributing the obituary of Tausk "to Freud himself." My reasons for including it in the Standard Edition are obvious. Although it had (in its original publication in the *Zeitschrift* in 1920) the vague subscription "Die Redaktion," nevertheless:
>
> First, it was included in the *Gesammelte Schriften*, over which Freud—despite his illness—exercised a general supervision.
>
> Second, it was included in the *Gesammelte Werke*, which was edited by persons in close touch with Freud.
>
> Third, the text of my translation, like all else, was sent to Anna Freud for her vetting before it was published, and I have before me evidence that she passed it without comment. I may say that she has always been very ready to question the authenticity of doubtful material.
>
> I have of course no knowledge of the weight of the critics quoted by you. Nor have I any reason to deny that the obituary may have been written by someone else (e.g., Rank) by Freud's instructions. But I think it is sensible to assume, in view of what I have said above, that it represents in general Freud's attitude.
>
> (J. Strachey, personal communication, January 28, 1967)

In the obituary, Freud praised Tausk's considerable psychoanalytic talent, as well as his impressive cultural and philosophical background. He emphasized that Tausk's promising career had been derailed by World War I, which subjected him to extreme economic and emotional hardship. Under such pressures, all intellectual productivity became fragmented and ultimately futile. Despite its brevity, this composition—arguably the longest obituary Freud ever wrote—concludes by affirming that Tausk would retain a significant place in the history of psychoanalysis, to which he had devoted himself wholeheartedly and whose cause he had never betrayed (Freud, 1919/1979g).

Nevertheless, Freud's explanation for Tausk's suicide appears overly reductive. He attributed the act primarily to the trauma of war, thereby overlooking deeper psychological, interpersonal, and institutional factors—perhaps in an effort to absolve both himself and the psychoanalytic community of responsibility (Guillerault, 1974). Freud's private reflections reveal a more conflicted and intimate perspective. Just three days after the suicide, on July 6, 1919, he informed Karl Abraham of Tausk's death, linking it retrospectively to a severe episode of vomiting and nervous agitation that Tausk had experienced during the most recent International Psychoanalytic Congress (Gay, 1988). Once again, Freud cited the war as a devastating influence that had left Tausk irreparably damaged.

In a letter dated July 10, 1919, addressed to Sándor Ferenczi—where he incorrectly dated the suicide to July 4—Freud interpreted the act through a psychoanalytic lens. He attributed it to psychic impotence and conceptualized it as the final manifestation of a childhood conflict with the paternal imago. The letter reads:

> Tausk shot himself on July 4, a week before the date set for his wedding, leaving behind tender and conciliatory letters. Etiology obscure, probably psychic impotence and the last act of his infantile struggle with the ghost of the father. Despite appreciation of his talent, no real sympathy in me.
>
> (Falzeder et al., 1996, p. 363)

Freud also conveyed news of the tragedy to Oskar Pfister (1873–1956), a Swiss Protestant pastor and long-standing proponent of psychoanalysis. In a letter dated July 13 of the same year, he described Tausk as a gifted man who ultimately succumbed to the burden of fate and the trauma of war (Freud & Pfister, 1963/1966). On August 1, Freud informed Lou Andreas-Salomé of Tausk's death, noting the affectionate tone and loyalty to psychoanalysis expressed in the farewell letter he had received. He speculated on the hidden motives that might have led his disciple to take such an irrevocable step. This letter—partially censored by Anna Freud in the first German edition of the correspondence between her father and Lou Andreas-Salomé (Freud & Andreas-Salomé, 1966/1968), ostensibly to protect Marius Tausk from emotional harm—can be reconstructed by comparing the redacted version with materials later published by Clark (1980/1985). It reads:

> The poor Tausk, whom you once honored with your friendship, deliberately ended his life on July 3. He returned from the war exhausted by its horrors, and in Vienna—under the most unfavorable conditions—had to rebuild the life disrupted by military service. He had sought to bring another woman into his life and was to be married in about eight days, but instead chose a different path.
>
> His farewell letters—to his fiancée, to his first wife, and to me—are all affectionate, clear, and free of blame toward anyone but himself, offering no real explanation for his final act. In his letter to me, he reaffirms his loyalty to psychoanalysis, thanks me, and so forth. But what lay beneath these words is impossible to discern [this portion comes from the uncensored version]. Deep down, he spent his life struggling against the paternal imago. I must admit I did not miss him; I had long understood that he would no longer be useful to us—or worse, that he might even become a future threat.
>
> I had already seen glimpses of the shaky foundations beneath his grandiose sublimations. I would have withdrawn from him much earlier had you not raised him so highly in my estimation. Of course, I was willing to help him advance, but at that point I could do very little, given the general collapse of circumstances in Vienna.
>
> I never denied his exceptional talents, but those were never matched by works of equal value.
>
> (Freud & Andreas-Salomé, 1966/1968, p. 129; Clark, 1980/1985, p. 215)

As previously noted—and as Roazen (1977) also confirmed—the first German edition of the Freud–Andreas-Salomé correspondence, which I consulted in its Spanish translation while preparing this book, omitted significant portions of this letter (Freud & Andreas-Salomé, 1966/1968). These omissions were subsequently corrected in the 1972 English edition, where the letter was published in its entirety. The complete text was later included as well in the second German edition of 1980 and in Binion's (1968) study of Lou Andreas-Salomé. According to Roazen (1972), Anna Freud's decision to censor the original letter stemmed less from concern for Marius Tausk's well-being than from a desire to safeguard her father's public image.

This editorial tendency was not unique to the case of Viktor Tausk; it appeared elsewhere as well—for instance, in Anna Freud's decision to withhold her father's critical comments about Alfred Adler in his correspondence with Arnold Zweig (1887–1968), the German-Jewish novelist and essayist who would later emerge as a distinguished voice in twentieth-century German literature. Of particular relevance to this study is a lesser-known episode involving the publication of Freud's correspondence with Lou Andreas-Salomé. The editorial responsibility for that volume lay with Ilse Grubrich-Simitis (1936–2024), in collaboration with Ernst Pfeiffer, and it was to her that Anna Freud addressed a significant letter regarding the inclusion of

Freud's statements about Tausk. In a letter dated July 17, 1966, Anna Freud requested that Grubrich-Simitis omit a particularly harsh passage in which her father, Sigmund Freud, spoke critically of Tausk—by then long deceased. The letter, later cited by Grubrich-Simitis herself (Grubrich-Simitis, 1991, p. 57), reads:

> [My father] speaks very openly, and in a derogatory and critical tone, about Dr. Tausk, who had by then already committed suicide. It is absolutely unnecessary to publish this part! I have just received a letter from his son, Marius Tausk, a professor in the Netherlands, asking to schedule an appointment. He wants me to tell him what my father [Sigmund Freud] thought of his. Clearly, the memory of his father—whom he lost at a very young age—continues to trouble him. I answered evasively, and when he comes, I will of course speak very cautiously. But if he were to read an assessment like the one my father gave, it could have very unpleasant consequences, which we must avoid at all costs. Would you please address this point with Pfeiffer? That would save me from having to write a second letter. Still, I would like to know, for my peace of mind, that there won't be a catastrophe.

Anna Freud's request to omit the harsh passage has been interpreted quite differently by Eissler. As he notes, its presence in the page proofs clearly indicates that no member of the Freud family had previously objected to its publication on the grounds that it might compromise Freud himself; otherwise, it would never have appeared there in the first place. According to Eissler, "It was consideration for the Tausk family that was the sole reason for that deletion" (Eissler, 1971, p. 18). I would argue, however, that while Anna's concern indeed reflects a protective impulse toward the surviving members of Viktor Tausk's family, it also reveals an implicit editorial posture—one intent on shaping the affective and reputational legacy of her father's private judgments. That Marius Tausk reached out to her personally underscores how emotionally charged and unresolved his father's fate remained, even decades later.

This moment—seemingly minor in editorial history—has broader implications. It reveals how tightly controlled the narrative surrounding Freud and his inner circle remained throughout the twentieth century, especially regarding contentious or ethically ambiguous episodes. Anna Freud's appeal to Ilse Grubrich-Simitis and Ernst Pfeiffer was more than a matter of editorial discretion; it was an effort to shape historical memory, particularly concerning a figure like Tausk, whose end cast a long and troubling shadow over the early psychoanalytic movement.

Such editorial interventions—motivated by a mix of ethical caution, filial loyalty, and reputational concern—remind me that the memory of Viktor Tausk has long been mediated through acts of discretion and omission. Yet amid this controlled legacy, I also find voices that speak with greater emotional candor. One such voice belongs to Lou Andreas-Salomé, whose correspondence with Freud reveals a markedly different tone: less defensive, more reflective—open to mourning rather than managing Tausk's memory.

In her reply dated August 25, Lou Andreas-Salomé expressed sorrow and surprise at Tausk's suicide, which she had not anticipated. She portrayed him as a man whose assertive exterior concealed a vulnerable, affectionate core—a complexity she regretted not having fully embraced:

> Your message came as a complete surprise. Poor Tausk! I cared for him. I believed I knew him, and yet I would never have imagined he would take his own life. (To me, a deliberately chosen death—not a threat or an attempt—signifies a form of health rather than illness). I do not know what method he used (as a physician, poison would have been readily available), but if he used a firearm, I can only imagine that his death represented the final, monstrous fulfillment of a kind of voluptuous pleasure—violent and passive at once. That was the essence of Tausk—his danger and his charm. In non-psychoanalytic terms, one might call it the soul of a beast with a tender heart. He knew I had reservations about him—my horror at his ambition to secure a professorship in Vienna. As recently as March, he still intended to visit Munich, which I strongly discouraged. I did not respond to his last letter—nor to many of the ones before. He was right when he wrote, a year ago: "No one sits at the table with a wretched man—not even you have done so." It's true. I didn't either. The one who will truly mourn him—and was likely the person he loved most deeply—is Jelka, his sister. I would like to write to her—if only I knew her address in Vienna or could recall her husband's name.
>
> (Freud & Andreas-Salomé, 1966/1968, p. 130)

On August 2, while vacationing in Badgastein, Freud sent a brief letter to Sabina Spielrein encouraging her to submit her manuscripts to a publisher, as he expected to be away throughout August and September. Whether Spielrein replied remains unknown. In this letter, Freud included a single, passing remark: "Dr. Tausk has ended his sad existence on July 3" (Carotenuto & Trombetta, 1981, p. 322).

In summary, regarding the suicide of Viktor Tausk—despite the inherent complexities involved in tracing the interplay of personal, clinical, and historical factors—it seems reasonable to suggest that his death might have been averted, or at least postponed. Freud possessed deep psychological insight into Tausk's character and had access to supplementary clinical observations from Helene Deutsch, who had conducted Tausk's analysis. Although Deutsch reported no signs of suicidal ideation during their three months of work, Freud's subsequent decision to compel her to choose between continuing her own treatment with him or maintaining her therapeutic relationship with Tausk placed Deutsch in an untenable position. This decision likely intensified Tausk's already significant narcissistic vulnerability, particularly his experience of rejection by the symbolic father. Such a rupture may have contributed—albeit in complex and indeterminate ways—to the psychic dynamics that ultimately culminated in his suicide.

As Roazen (1990, p. 133) poignantly observed, perhaps Tausk's suicide represented an unconscious attempt to avoid "killing" Freud—a tragic enactment of the ambivalence that defined their intensely charged relationship. This interpretation underscores how profoundly their bond exceeded the ordinary contours of an analytic or collegial connection. What bound them was not merely intellectual affinity but a deep emotional entanglement, woven from dependency, idealization, rivalry, and unrelenting ambivalence.

In stark contrast, Eissler (1971) adopts a markedly dismissive and scornful stance toward Tausk. He argues that Tausk was merely "an accident in Freud's life," asserting that Freud's personal and intellectual development would have remained essentially unchanged had Tausk stayed in Berlin and never entered his circle. Furthermore, Eissler reduces Tausk's legacy to "little more than a reflection of Freud" in the eyes of posterity (p. 190).

This unequivocal alignment with Freud's legacy—at the expense of Tausk—strikes me as excessive, and somewhat improper for a scholar of Eissler's seriousness. In this instance, he seems to exceed the prudent limits of academic critique, adopting a hagiographic posture in defense of Freud while diminishing Tausk to a mere shadow of his mentor. Such a stance risks obscuring the tragic singularity of Tausk's trajectory and underestimates the complexity of his psychological reality.

It is important to acknowledge, however, that Eissler (1971, p. 190) somewhat tempers his earlier harshness in the same passage, conceding:

> Tausk was talented in his own right, of course, and it is conceivable that he might have acquired some degree of prestige as a journalist. By many reasons could be adduced that make it probable that the profession of journalism would have harbored grave dangers for such a personality as Tausk's. It is a moot question.

Moreover, Eissler continues: "The fact is that Freud was bound to attract disciples, and one cannot therefore ascribe to any one of them individually the role or function of either protagonist or antagonist necessary to his rise" (Eissler, 1971, p. 190).

This acknowledgment does little to soften the severity of Eissler's earlier judgment, yet it introduces a more nuanced perspective—one that refuses to reduce Tausk solely to a subordinate figure within Freud's orbit. By recognizing Tausk's individual talents and the complex relational dynamics of Freud's early circle, Eissler implicitly opens a space for reconsidering Tausk not merely as an accessory to Freud's legacy, but as a figure worthy of independent recognition.

From my perspective as a historian of psychoanalysis, such balance is essential. It is crucial to resist reductive narratives that risk eclipsing the multifaceted nature of Tausk's contributions and the profound psychological struggles that shaped both his life and work. Only through this measured lens can we begin to grasp the full scope of his tragic trajectory without diminishing his singularity or the historical significance of his psychoanalytic insights.

Building upon this more nuanced and psychoanalytic perspective, Tausk's suicide can be understood as the tragic culmination of a life deeply marked by what appears to have been a severe narcissistic personality disorder. He suffered from chronic dysthymic states permeated by guilt—likely rooted not only in genetic predispositions but also in a profoundly disturbed early affective environment. This formative context seems to have fostered ambivalent object relations, characterized by overt hostility toward the paternal figure alongside simultaneous identification with him. In parallel, his relationship with the maternal figure—and with women in general—was marked by sadomasochistic dynamics.

In his search for a substitute paternal figure, Tausk became entangled in a neurotically charged and mutually neurotizing relationship with Freud. This dynamic—saturated with idealization and dependency on Tausk's part, and with distancing and mistrust on Freud's—may have been pivotal in precipitating the tragic denouement. For Tausk, the experience of what he likely perceived as ultimate failure—the absence of acceptance or love from his symbolic father—may have been unbearably devastating. Nonetheless, it is important to recognize that Tausk's relationship with authority was not uniformly destructive. As discussed earlier, his defiance of established power structures was also animated by a profound ethical sensibility. This moral dimension is exemplified in his courageous advocacy for wartime deserters, whose lives he saved through interventions made possible by his rare combination of legal training and psychiatric expertise—having served both as a judge and as a physician.

Clinically, Tausk's psychic landscape appears to have been shaped by a profound narcissistic disturbance, characterized by intense aggressive tendencies—particularly in the sexual realm—interwoven with pervasive guilt and persecutory anxiety, the latter perhaps arising from the projection of his own hostility. His inner world bore the heavy burden of narcissistic dysthymia, manifesting in recurrent feelings of impotence and hopelessness in the face of ideals forever beyond reach. These conflicts were compounded by significant ego-function deficits, especially in his capacity to sustain balanced and enduring interpersonal relationships.

Superimposed upon these features were patterns of histrionic manipulation and unresolved difficulties in separation–individuation, supported only by the fragile scaffolding of a self-esteem oscillating between devaluation, the lash of a harsh and persecutory superego, and grandiose ambitions unmoored from the realities of his actual achievements. Taken together, this clinical configuration resonates closely with the conceptualization advanced by Bleichmar (1997), whose formulation of narcissistic pathology continues to offer a compelling lens through which to illuminate the tragic arc of Tausk's existence.

With these clinical considerations, I approach the close of my psychoanalytic portrait of Viktor Tausk—a portrait I will bring to completion in the following chapter through a detailed analysis of his technical writings. At this point, I begin to set aside the man himself, leaving behind the living, suffering being, to allow his texts, at last, to speak on his behalf.

And yet, however carefully one might diagnose his inner wounds, such readings cannot—and must not—be allowed to diminish the originality or enduring value of Tausk's contributions to psychoanalysis. To judge an author's thought exclusively through the prism of his psychopathology risks collapsing the necessary distinction between the individual and the ideas he has bequeathed us. For this reason, I prefer to leave open a space in which each reader may encounter Tausk's writings on their own terms—unencumbered by reductive interpretations—allowing his voice to emerge before any final verdict is rendered. In this way, the reader is invited to weigh for themselves the depth, originality, and lasting resonance of his thought: to see not only the man who suffered, but also the analyst who dared to think.

Chapter 5

The Psychoanalytic Work of Viktor Tausk

A Promising but Truncated Body of Work

Viktor Tausk was not, by any measure, a prolific author. He left behind no books, only a small corpus of articles, lectures, and significant interventions delivered at the Vienna Psychoanalytic Society between 1909—when he was first admitted as a member—and his final contribution on March 31, 1915, as recorded in the official *Minutes of the Vienna Psychoanalytic Society* (Nunberg & Federn, 1967, 1974, 1975). Yet within this modest body of work resides the imprint of a mind of remarkable breadth and originality. His psychoanalytic writings—both oral and written—reveal an intellect of wide-ranging curiosity, endowed with a fervent desire for understanding and an unwavering ethical commitment to the alleviation of psychological suffering.

At the time of his death, Tausk was reportedly working on a *psychiatry manual*—a project that, had it survived, might well have secured his place among the most innovative thinkers of the early psychoanalytic movement. In one of his final gestures, however, he instructed that all his personal papers, letters, and manuscripts be destroyed unread. His younger son, Victor Hugo, fulfilled this last wish with filial devotion, reportedly spending an entire day carrying out the task. Through this act of erasure, Tausk seemed to vanish twice over: first as a man, through suicide; then as a psychoanalyst, through the annihilation of his unfinished intellectual legacy.

Despite this irreparable loss, one work survived to ensure his lasting place in psychoanalytic history: the seminal essay "On the origin of the 'influencing machine' in schizophrenia" (Tausk, 1919/1983a). Presented to the Vienna Psychoanalytic Society in 1918—though curiously absent from the official minutes—it stands as a cornerstone in the psychoanalytic understanding of psychosis. Prior to this, and apart from Freud's "Psycho-analytic notes on an autobiographical account of a case of paranoia (dementia paranoides)" (Freud, 1911/1980b), only Jung had attempted a comparable application of psychoanalytic concepts to the psychoses. This early line of inquiry would later be expanded by figures such as Paul Federn, Harry Stack Sullivan (1892–1949), Bruno Bettelheim (1903–1990), and Erik Homburger Erikson (1902–1994) (Roazen, 1972, 1990).

DOI: 10.4324/9781003716426-5

Among these successors, Paul Federn stands out as a pivotal figure in the second generation of Freudians. His work on ego psychology—particularly his exploration of the ego's boundaries and their disturbances in schizophrenia—became central to the post-Freudian development of clinical theory (Weiss, 1991). Yet this very concept, which later became synonymous with Federn's name, is historically and ethically entangled with Tausk's intellectual legacy. Federn never publicly acknowledged Tausk as the originator of the idea of the *ego boundary* and even went so far as to accuse him of plagiarism. This claim, however, was quietly overturned after Federn's death: in an obituary published in *Psychoanalytic Quarterly*, Bertram D. Lewin (1950) explicitly affirmed that the foundational notion of the ego boundary had, in fact, originated with Tausk (p. 296).

Still, uncertainty persists. Weiss (1991) cautiously admitted that it remains unclear whether Tausk or Federn first coined the term *Ichgrenze* (ego boundary), though he maintained that Federn achieved a more fully elaborated understanding of ego psychology in his later writings (p. 11). By contrast, Roazen (2005) asserted unequivocally that Tausk was the first to develop both the concepts of identity and ego boundaries, preceding Federn's formulation. As Roazen explained, Tausk's theoretical innovation lay in emphasizing that psychological illness could arise not from an excess of instinctual energy—as Freud posited—but from a *deficiency* in ego strength, a fragility that left the psyche vulnerable and in need of external support (p. 131).

To clarify this historical issue, I corresponded for many years with Ernst Federn—Paul Federn's son and the faithful custodian of his father's legacy—between 1999 and his death in 2007, as previously discussed in Chapter 2. In a letter dated March 10, 2000, Ernst wrote to me that "it is impossible to find out who created the term 'ego boundaries'" (E. Federn, personal communication, March 10, 2000). One year later, on December 6, 2001, he deepened his reflection with an observation of great significance: "Tausk was the first to consider the weak ego in his famous paper of 1919. He was a friend of my father, and we do not know who first observed the lack of cathexis in the mentally ill" (E. Federn, personal communication, December 6, 2001).

The conceptual lineage that began with Tausk was soon extended by Helene Deutsch, whose paper "Ein kasuistischer Beitrag zur Kenntnis des Mechanismus der Regression bei Schizophrenie" [A case-based contribution to the understanding of the mechanism of regression in schizophrenia] (Deutsch, 1919) was submitted as part of her formal application to the Vienna Psychoanalytic Society. The paper later appeared in English under the modified title "A case that throws light on the mechanism of regression in schizophrenia" (Deutsch & Roazen, 1985; Roazen, 1992, pp. 164–165). The mark of Tausk's thinking can thus be traced not only in the development of psychoanalytic theory but also in the institutional evolution of the movement itself—particularly in its growing willingness to engage with the complexities of psychotic experience.

Within this trajectory, and as has been mentioned earlier, Tausk's essay "On the origin of the 'influencing machine' in schizophrenia" (Tausk, 1919/1983a) remains a landmark, extending Freud's theoretical edifice into a territory long considered resistant to psychoanalytic inquiry. If Freud's 1911 analysis of the Schreber case inaugurated the psychoanalytic approach to paranoia (Freud, 1911/1980b), Tausk's contribution carried this endeavor further—into the phenomenology of schizophrenia. His paper offered one of the earliest and most penetrating psychoanalytic interpretations of delusional systems, an interpretive leap that bridged the chasm between descriptive psychiatry and dynamic psychology.

Interwoven with this exploration of psychosis was Tausk's deep and sustained interest in narcissism—a theme that pervades his theoretical reflections and clinical practice alike. Decades later, Hanns Sachs would echo some of these concerns in "The delay of the machine age" (Sachs, 1933), a work that has remained relatively neglected within the psychoanalytic canon but which deserves renewed attention. In Section 4 of his essay, Sachs traced the historical development of human creativity, suggesting that early humanity's fusion with the bodily ego—and a primitive form of narcissism—posed significant obstacles to technological innovation (Moellenhoff, 1966/1968).

Sachs also ventured into the affective and intrapsychic dimensions of aesthetic experience, proposing a subtle kinship between the experience of beauty and that of sadness. Beauty, in his account, emerges not as a static quality but as a transformation of affect—an achievement of sublimation that binds mourning and creation in a single psychic act.

Among Tausk's posthumously published works, one article—long believed lost—resurfaced unexpectedly in 1934: "Ibsen the druggist." It first appeared in German in the *Almanach der Psychoanalyse, 9,* pp. 161–166 under the title "Psychopathologie des Alltagslebens: Ibsen, der Apotheker" [Psychopathology of everyday life: Ibsen the druggist] (Tausk, 1934a) and was later translated into English by Dorian Feigenbaum, abbreviated only as "Ibsen the druggist," and published in *Psychoanalytic Quarterly*, 3(1), pp. 137–141 (Tausk, 1934b; Roazen, 2017a, pp. 221–225). Interestingly, in the Spanish edition of Tausk's collected works, the same essay appears under the title "Contribution to the psychology of everyday life" (Tausk, 1934/1983a, pp. 223–227)—a discrepancy already noted earlier in this book.

As Roazen (1990) observed, the true significance of this article lies less in its explicit content than in its latent meaning. Beneath its surface, "Ibsen the druggist" can be read as a veiled, autobiographical meditation on Tausk's inner conflicts and his ambivalent relationship with Freud. In this sense, the essay stands as both a theoretical contribution and a personal testament—an echo of the unresolved psychic tensions that shaped the tragic and incandescent trajectory of Viktor Tausk's brief intellectual life.

Contributions to the Study of Sexuality

Viktor Tausk's first publication on the subject of sexuality, "On masturbation" (Tausk, 1912/1983a), addressed a topic that had long preoccupied the Vienna Psychoanalytic Society, which devoted a series of meetings to its discussion. As detailed in Chapter 4 of this book, the Society's first scientific session on masturbation took place on November 22, 1911—a moment that marked a significant stage in Tausk's intellectual integration into Freud's circle.

The collected contributions from those sessions were later published under the title *Die Onanie: Vierzehn Beiträge zu einer Diskussion der Wiener Psychoanalytischen Vereinigung* [Masturbation: Fourteen contributions to a discussion of the Vienna Psychoanalytic Society] (Die Onanie, 1912; Nunberg & Federn, 1974, p. 320). Many of the interventions recorded in the *Minutes*—analyzed earlier in this volume—illustrate the seriousness with which masturbation was treated, not as a moral question but as a complex psychological and developmental phenomenon.

In his essay, based on clinical observations of 18 patients, Tausk approaches masturbation not merely as a solitary sexual act but as a symbolic expression shaped by the psychic and affective meanings attributed to it by the subject. Fully attuned to the subtlety and richness of this terrain, he organizes his analysis according to four interrelated criteria: *propensity, causes, motives and forms*, and *purposes and effects*. He defines masturbation as a sexual activity—whether involving the genitals or a secondary erogenous zone—that dispenses with a partner and aims at the direct relief of sexual tension. Crucially, he identifies accompanying fantasy as the defining element of the act, for it discloses its essential psychic structure.

From this premise, Tausk isolates a particularly illuminating variant, which he terms *psychic masturbation*: the discharge of sexual excitation through fantasy alone, without any preceding somatic stimulation. He interprets this form as an expression of the child's incestuous object choices, which may involve both animate and inanimate objects, and may be directed toward either sex. Regarding homosexual fantasies, Tausk observes that children tend to abandon such content around the ages of 5 or 6—a developmental transition he interprets as signaling the establishment of a heterosexual orientation.

Perhaps the most original and penetrating aspect of Tausk's paper lies in his understanding of *adolescent masturbation*. He conceives of it as a provisional mode of satisfaction whose function is to prolong childhood artificially—a psychic strategy conditioned by prevailing social and moral prohibitions. In deterring the adolescent from initiating coital relations, masturbation sustains a fixation on autoerotic pleasure and thereby delays emotional maturation.

According to Tausk, the latency period of puberty—characterized by the inhibition of overt sexual gratification—serves two fundamental functions. The first, *pedagogical*, allows for ego development and socialization through the temporary detachment of the ego from its somatic basis. The second, *biological*, facilitates the renunciation of masturbation in favor of object choice and reproductive aims. Yet this developmental trajectory is disrupted by a double moral bind: society denies adolescents authentic genital experience with a partner while simultaneously condemning masturbation as a regressive act. The adolescent thus becomes psychically entrapped between instinctual demand and cultural interdiction, a conflict that may provoke regression to earlier psychosexual stages and reanimate oedipal fixations. The intensification of the oedipal struggle, in turn, threatens the consolidation of genital sexuality, which for Tausk represents the culmination of sexual development.

Tausk also investigates the physiological and psychological consequences of masturbation, exploring the struggle against habituation and the ambivalent attitudes it generates. Physically, he concurs with other contemporary authorities in affirming that moderate masturbation is not harmful and may even yield benefits. He addresses nocturnal emissions, rejecting Freud's early theory that linked them inherently to neurotic symptoms. While acknowledging that excessive frequency might weaken the nervous or secretory systems, he considers such hypotheses largely obsolete.

Psychologically, Tausk highlights anxiety, guilt, disturbances in object choice, and submissive attitudes toward authority as its principal outcomes. Anxiety, in his view, constitutes the central affective consequence of masturbation, arising either from an incomplete libidinal discharge—a quantitative failure—or from insufficient means of release—a qualitative defect. In this respect, Tausk remains consistent with Freud's first theory of anxiety, which associated the symptom with the accumulation of unexpended libido.

He then asks under what conditions an individual may achieve sexual fulfillment in adulthood after engaging in masturbatory activity during adolescence. The determining factors, he proposes, are the maturity of object libido and the degree to which infantile perversions have been gratified through autoerotic means. Should the libido remain fixated at an infantile level, the subject may persist in masturbation as the sole mode of discharge—thereby avoiding anxiety but precluding mature satisfaction. Such persistence, he argues, predisposes the individual to neurosis. Moreover, when masturbatory fantasies involve perversions that cannot be symbolically or perceptually satisfied—such as olfactory perversions in the absence of hallucinatory capacity—the inevitable result is frustration.

Regarding guilt, Tausk offers a subtle formulation: it emerges only in those for whom masturbation fails to yield full satisfaction; in those who achieve it, guilt is absent. Here, moral conflict is revealed as a symptom of psychic incompleteness rather than transgression per se.

In considering *object choice*, Tausk maintains that masturbation delays the formation of genuine interpersonal relationships, since the act remains narcissistically self-referential. The masturbator avoids both the internal imperative of species preservation and the external demand for relational engagement. This dual evasion intensifies moral condemnation, deepening psychic conflict. Trapped between instinctual drive and social prohibition, the subject may lose interest in reciprocal intimacy, reducing coitus to a mere continuation of solitary pleasure. Within this dynamic, fantasy becomes paramount: a hallucinatory substitute for emotional connection. If such a pattern becomes fixed, the individual may drift toward neurosis or a homosexual fixation, insofar as all erotic investment remains closed within the self.

In Tausk's clinical practice, numerous male patients reported overcoming masturbation through heterosexual intercourse; yet many, he observed, reduced their partners to mere instruments of gratification. For these men, coitus itself degenerated into a form of *masturbatory coitus*—a relational façade concealing psychic isolation. Lacking empathy and mutual attunement, they approached sexuality through fantasy rather than through encounter. The result was chronic frustration and impotence, often leading them toward prostitution, where eroticism and tenderness were forcibly split. Tausk identifies the cynicism that frequently follows such experiences as a rationalized defense—a mask for emotional disillusionment and the failure to integrate tenderness and desire.

In conclusion, Tausk characterizes masturbation as the convergence of three destructive forces: first, it undermines self-esteem by eroding the subject's sense of sexual and relational competence; second, it reinforces immaturity, weakening the individual's authority in familial and social spheres; and third, it diminishes virility—not only physiologically, through premature stimulation, but also affectively, by inhibiting mutual fulfillment and generating frustration in partners.

While acknowledging the role of constitutional factors, Tausk attributes decisive weight to environmental influences—especially to familial and educational practices. He condemns traditional pedagogies that repress children's spontaneous access to sexual knowledge and experience. According to his analysis, the renunciation of masturbation coincides with the resolution of unconscious sadism toward the father; when adolescents are forcibly infantilized by an authoritarian culture, masturbation re-emerges as an act of rebellion—a symbolic emancipation from paternal impotence. Tausk closes with a lament for the pedagogical indifference of educators to the sexual life of youth: deprived of adequate guidance, adolescents remain trapped in bodily pleasure and passive dependence, unable to achieve reciprocal, embodied sexuality.

Fourteen years later, Wilhelm Reich (1897–1957) would revisit many of these themes in his essay "Parents as educators: The compulsion to educate and its causes" (Reich, 1926/1984), originally published in German as "Eltern als Erzieher: I. Der Erziehungszwang und seine Ursachen" in the *Zeitschrift für Psychoanalytische Pädagogik, 1*(*3*), 65–74. Reich reformulated Tausk's insights within a more explicitly social and political frame, transforming psychoanalytic reflection into the groundwork for institutional innovation, including the establishment of sexual-hygiene clinics—a decisive step from interpretation to praxis.

Tausk's subsequent major contribution to the study of sexuality, "Contribution to the psychology of infantile sexuality" (Tausk, 1913c/1983a), opens with a meditation on the pervasive repression and hypocrisy surrounding sexuality in modern culture. This moral climate, he argues, impedes direct clinical access to children's sexual experiences, compelling the analyst to seek indirect routes of inquiry. He thus turns to dream analysis as a privileged methodological instrument. In this context, he presents a series of dreams narrated by a 10-year-old boy named Fritz, with whom he felt a strong personal affinity—an affective bond that, he believed, deepened his interpretive understanding. As Kanzer (1971) later observed, the child in question was in fact Marius Tausk, the author's eldest son—a detail confirmed by Marius himself (M. Tausk, 1973).

Drawing on this material, Tausk offers a pointed critique of Alfred Adler's theory of the *masculine protest*, rejecting the view that the desire to be male arises primarily from social comparison and the will to power. Instead, he situates it within the intrapsychic sphere, as a conflict between competing instinctual trends—a dialectic internal to the libido rather than a product of cultural valuation (Tausk, 1913c/1983a). He further observes that the sexual life of children in the latency period is dominated by voyeuristic curiosity, particularly fascination with the intimate hygiene habits of others. This observational drive, assimilated later through familial and educational experience, provides the raw material for adolescent sexual fantasies.

Tausk's final significant contribution to the psychoanalytic study of sexuality appears in his commentary on Karl Abraham's paper on "ejaculatio praecox" (Tausk, 1917/1983a), itself written in response to two earlier essays—Ferenczi's "On the significance of 'ejaculatio praecox'" (Ferenczi, 1908/1981a) and Abraham's own study of 1917 (Abraham, 1917/1994). Ferenczi's pioneering work is particularly notable for its advocacy of women's sexual rights, especially their right to orgasmic fulfillment, which he regarded as obstructed not by biological factors but by culture—by the asymmetrical moral order that sanctioned male premarital experience while condemning female sexuality. Although Ferenczi admitted his limited understanding of the sociological forces underpinning this double standard, he nonetheless linked women's sexual emancipation to a potential decline in hysteria, envisioning an equilibrium between repression and excessive liberation. He perceived in contemporary debates on women's sexual initiation the early signs of such transformation, warning that without change, male sexual dysfunction and female anesthesia might perpetuate themselves across generations—a kind of quasi-Lamarckian inheritance of repression.

A few years later, Wilhelm Reich (1921–1922) would revisit these issues in his essay "Der Koitus und die Geschlechter" [Coition and the sexes], where he opposed Karl Urbach's claim that the female orgasm was merely secondary to the male's. Urbach, then a *cand. med.* (candidate of medicine), had advanced this view in his article "Über die zeitliche Gefühlsdifferenz während der Kohabitation" [On the temporal difference of feelings during coitus] (Urbach, 1921–1922, pp. 124–138), published in the same volume (*Zeitschrift für Sexualwissenschaft, 8*) that would later include Reich's own reply (Reich, 1921–1922, pp. 343–352). In his opening remarks, Reich explicitly cited Urbach's paper from the July 1921 issue, situating his critique within the ongoing debate on sexual asymmetry.

Reich's intervention marked a decisive departure from the biologically reductionist assumptions underlying Urbach's argument. Rather than viewing sexual difference as an immutable physiological fact, he interpreted it as the outcome of cultural repression and moral conditioning. In doing so, Reich relocated the question of erotic disparity from the body to the psyche, opening the way toward a more dynamic understanding of sexual experience as both an intrapsychic and social phenomenon.

Returning, then, to Abraham's own essay (Abraham, 1917/1994), he introduced a novel framework for understanding *ejaculatio praecox*, identifying two defining elements: premature seminal emission and a series of non-rhythmic muscular contractions—phenomena that, in his view, rendered the act more analogous to urination than to mature sexual release. He traced the dysfunction to a fixation on urethral erotism, a residual pleasure associated with urination that obstructs the full transition to genital organization. His clinical observations supported this thesis: patients frequently exhibited diminished sensitivity of the glans and heightened responsiveness in the perineum and posterior scrotum—zones homologous to the female vaginal entrance. Abraham thus concluded that *ejaculatio praecox* signaled an incomplete consolidation of the masculine sexual organization.

Extending this logic, Abraham proposed a striking analogy between male *ejaculatio praecox* and female frigidity. In both, he saw a restriction of erotic gratification to secondary erogenous zones—the urethra and clitoris—signaling a regression toward the dominant zone of the opposite sex. The result, he argued, was a partial, pregenital organization of sexuality.

Tausk's response was incisive and critical. He questioned whether Abraham's analogy could stand unless frigidity were demonstrably linked to intensified urethral erotism in women. He further doubted that female frigidity could always be interpreted through urethral fixation, particularly in cases where arousal occurred through other erogenous zones. He also noted that Abraham's etiological parallel was inconsistent: if both conditions derived from a shared fixation, they should exhibit homologous features—yet Abraham did not establish this. Finally, Tausk pointed out that Abraham avoided the most consequential implication of his own logic: if fixation on the erogenous zone of the opposite sex indicates a homosexual component, this should be explicitly acknowledged—especially in light of the extensive psychoanalytic literature linking homosexuality and impotence.

In place of Abraham's schema, Tausk offered alternative hypotheses, some drawn from Abraham's earlier insights. He suggested that premature ejaculation might express a narcissistic refusal to relinquish semen, akin to Abraham's notion of fecal retention as a manifestation of emotional stinginess. The man who withholds, Tausk argued, loves his partner in appearance while unconsciously giving nothing. He also proposed that *ejaculatio praecox* may encode unconscious hostility toward women: the woman excites desire but simultaneously evokes resentment or unworthiness. This ambivalence, intolerable to consciousness, is acted out through the abbreviation of the sexual act, which thereby assumes sadistic coloring.

The compulsive urgency to "empty oneself," in Tausk's reading, signifies a psychic retreat—an escape from the anxiety of fusion or loss. For men burdened by intense castration anxiety, the premature ending of the sexual act serves as a defensive maneuver: the preservation of autonomy through the avoidance of surrender. Conversely, Tausk noted cases of the opposite symptom—an inability to ejaculate—interpreting them as manifestations of psychic paralysis and emotional self-containment. In both instances, he discerned the same underlying disturbance: a narcissistic withdrawal that leaves the female partner feeling frustrated, abandoned, and unmet—a clinical constellation that, as Abraham himself had observed, reveals the enduring fragility of love when shadowed by narcissism.

A Psychoanalytic Approach to Psychosis

In addressing this fascinating and clinically significant topic—one that continues to captivate psychoanalytic and neuroscientific inquiry alike, particularly concerning its origins, course, outcomes, and possibilities for treatment—I turn to Viktor Tausk's incisive study, "On the psychology of alcoholic occupational delirium" (Tausk, 1915/1983a). Drawing on a series of cases from Wagner-Jauregg's clinic, Tausk explores an original and revealing analogy between alcoholic occupational delirium—a condition marked by compulsive, purposeless labor during altered states of consciousness—and dreams in which the dreamer performs incomplete or futile tasks. The distinction he draws is subtle yet profound: in occupational delirium, the subject is consumed by monotonous, repetitive labor devoid of satisfaction, whereas in dreams, though the structure may be similar, the activity is not necessarily tinged with futility or distress. What unites both phenomena is the inescapable presence of anxiety that accompanies the act of "working."

This analogy—first suggested to Tausk by his colleague, the medical student Fräulein Ilse Zimmermann (Tausk, 1915/1983a, p. 46)—was received with skepticism by those who resisted applying psychoanalytic reasoning to psychoses of organic origin. To such critics, the cerebral lesion itself was explanation enough. Tausk, however, challenged this reductionism, arguing that purely neurological accounts could not capture the subtle variations in symptom expression and meaning that emerge in the lived experience of alcoholic patients.

The originality of his view became evident during the scientific meeting of March 31, 1915, at the Vienna Psychoanalytic Society, where his paper sparked intense discussion (Nunberg & Federn, 1975, pp. 288–292). Particularly striking was the moment when Tausk referred to the symbolic dimension of the dream motif of *working*—an interpretation first formulated by Hans Sperber (1885–1963). In his study "Über den Einfluß sexueller Momente auf Entstehung und Entwicklung der Sprache" [On the influence of sexual factors on the origin and development of language] (*Imago, 1*, 405–453), Sperber (1912) proposed that the repetitive, quasi-mechanical activities of early human labor were infused with libidinal meaning, shaping both language and symbolic thought. Tausk adopted this premise to interpret dreams of endless, uncompleted tasks as expressions of impotence—both literal and symbolic—analogous to the restless, automatic labor of alcoholic delirium. He suggested that these dreams represent an unconscious dramatization of dissatisfaction born of sexual abstinence, a psychic state in which the partner is reduced to a mere instrument of pleasure, exposing the narcissistic and homosexual undercurrents of the subject's psychic structure.

Kanzer (1971) later speculated that Tausk's clinical vignette of a 23-year-old philology student suffering from impotence might conceal an autobiographical confession. Marius Tausk (1973), however, vehemently denied this claim, emphasizing his father's moral integrity and professional rigor. Yet Kanzer (1973a) remained unconvinced—a controversy that, while anecdotal, underscores the enduring transference of fascination and ambivalence surrounding Tausk's figure.

The work that ultimately secured Tausk's place in psychoanalytic history was "On the origin of the 'influencing machine' in schizophrenia" (Tausk, 1919/1983a). In this study—based on a single clinical case—Tausk left behind the domain of organic psychosis to enter the symbolic universe of functional psychotic states. As Grotjahn and Illing (1966/1968) observed, it is exceedingly rare for one essay to establish a permanent reputation in psychoanalysis; Tausk's may be the exception. The essay was later anthologized by Robert Fliess in *The Psychoanalytic Reader* (Fliess, 1948), translated into English in 1933 in *Psychoanalytic Quarterly, 2*, 519–556, and into Spanish in 1945 in *Revista de Psicoanálisis, 2(3)*, 490–524, thereby securing its canonical place within the psychoanalytic corpus.

In this landmark text, Tausk describes a striking delusional formation commonly found among schizophrenic patients: the *influencing machine.* Although patients seldom provide a complete description, their accounts share recurring imagery—a mechanical apparatus composed of wires, wheels, batteries, and gears, emitting rays or currents that govern their sensations, movements, and thoughts. The machine thus becomes the explanatory core of a vast delusional system, giving form to what might otherwise remain a formless chaos of internal experience.

Tausk's originality lies in refusing to treat these as isolated symptoms. Instead, he integrates them into a unified psychic structure. Patients often report seeing projected images, not in three dimensions but as flat, lantern-slide projections cast by the machine. They believe their thoughts and emotions are inserted or stolen by external forces, and that involuntary bodily events—such as erections or emissions—are caused by the machine's assault on their sexuality. Even tactile or visceral sensations, for which no ordinary language exists, are attributed to its workings. Through this imaginative construction, the patient externalizes and organizes experiences that have become intolerably alien within the self.

One of Tausk's most compelling cases is that of Natalia A., a 31-year-old former philosophy student who became deaf after a severe ear infection. Convinced that she had been under the influence of an electrical apparatus for more than six years, she claimed the device—illegally constructed in Berlin—was modeled after her own body and exerted power not only over her but over her mother as well. After rejecting a suitor, she believed that he, unable to win her affection, had turned to technological domination, employing the machine to manipulate her emotions and even her relationships.

For Tausk (1919/1983a), this delusional structure represents a projection of the patient's own bodily organs—most notably the genitals—transformed into a persecutory mechanism. The refusal to recognize the machine as part of the self is a desperate psychic defense that preserves ego coherence by disavowing the threatening source of inner conflict. Natalia's dreams of decapitated figures, symbolizing a radical loss of identity and corporeal integrity, reinforce this reading: the mechanical imagery constitutes a further step in the depersonalization and de-eroticization of the self.

From this foundation, Tausk proposed a developmental sequence of ego-boundary formation: first, an initial phase of undifferentiated unity between self and world; second, a phase in which projection establishes psychic separateness; and third, the emergence of a stable ego capable of distinguishing internal from external reality. Within this model, narcissism plays a central role. Tausk differentiates between innate and acquired narcissism and distinguishes normal from pathological projection. As he writes:

> Projection in early normal development arises because the innate narcissistic libidinal position is abandoned in response to external excitations; pathological projection, by contrast, emerges from an accumulation of narcissistic libido—primitive, regressive, or residual. This libido retains the qualities of innate narcissism: it excludes the subject from the external world. The projection of the body, therefore, defends against a libidinal position corresponding to the end of fetal life and the beginning of extrauterine existence. (Tausk, 1919/1983a, p. 208)

These insights would also inform Tausk's understanding of melancholia, which he conceived as a collapse of the narcissistic structure resulting from the ego's withdrawal of self-love. He had already elaborated these ideas in his lecture "Contributions to a psychoanalytic exposition of melancholia," delivered on December 30, 1914, before an audience of his psychoanalytic colleagues (Nunberg & Federn, 1975, pp. 272–276). Later, he encountered Freud's "Mourning and melancholia" (Freud, 1917/1979f), whose conceptual parallels reveal a shared trajectory of thought.

Refining the psychodynamics of schizophrenia, Tausk (1919/1983a) identified a triadic relational structure within the delusion: persecutors, persecuted, and emotionally significant figures—often maternal or medical—who remain exempt from hostility and serve as repositories of libidinal investment. Yet, figures of romantic interest evoke defensive aggression; affection is experienced as a threat to narcissistic integrity, prompting the erection of delusional defenses.

Thus, the *influencing machine* is not merely a product of psychotic disorganization but a regressive dramatization of the struggle between object libido and narcissistic libido. Any external object that demands libidinal investment—regardless of gender—becomes both coveted and feared, evoking ambivalence, suspicion, and hostility. The delusion therefore serves a paradoxical function: it both externalizes unbearable inner conflict and preserves psychic cohesion at the brink of fragmentation.

Later commentators, particularly Orange et al. (1997), deepened this understanding by situating the phenomenon within an intersubjective framework. Building on Tausk's insight that schizophrenia entails a "loss of ego boundaries" (p. 56), they describe the delusion not merely as projection but as a collapse of the geometry of subjective space itself. The machine's locus is unstable—at once inside and outside the self—while the constant is the lived sense of being *influenced*, of one's agency having been usurped.

From this perspective, the delusion crystallizes within relational contexts of profound submission, where personal initiative has been supplanted by alien will. The sexualized imagery of rays, penetration, and mechanical violation is not to be read as latent eroticism but as a symbolic expression of psychic violation—a "rape of the mind." By giving concrete form to an otherwise diffuse terror, the machine becomes paradoxically protective: an object that can be located, resisted, or destroyed.

In this way, Tausk's intrapsychic model and the intersubjective revisions that followed converge: both reveal the delusion as a creative act of survival, a last-ditch effort of the psyche to preserve coherence and meaning in the face of disintegration.

Interest in the Psychology of the Deserter

In his essay "On the psychology of the war deserter" (Tausk, 1916c/1983a), Viktor Tausk offers one of the earliest psychoanalytic explorations of a phenomenon that straddles the boundary between law, morality, and psychopathology: the act of desertion. This study, grounded in Tausk's wartime clinical experience, is remarkable not only for its depth of psychological insight but also because it represents the first time psychoanalysis entered what would later become the field of forensic psychology—a domain to which Sándor Ferenczi would subsequently make significant contributions.

Tausk begins by acknowledging the immense complexity of assessing legal responsibility in cases of desertion, given the often-fatal consequences of such acts. He insists that any adequate understanding must transcend juridical and moral judgments, requiring instead both a diachronic and synchronic analysis of the phenomenon—that is, one attentive to its psychological, historical, and institutional determinants. At the center of his argument lies a critique of military legislation, which he regards as outdated, one-dimensional, and insufficiently attuned to the unconscious forces shaping human conduct. Law, in his view, errs gravely when it presumes that behavior can be fully explained in terms of conscious intention.

Rejecting the conventional view that deserters are simply cowards or deliberate offenders, Tausk reframes desertion as a symptom of psychic distress—a compromise formation expressing conflict between duty and unconscious impulses. He develops a nuanced typology to capture the diversity of unconscious motivations underlying this act. Some deserters, he observes, flee under conditions of altered consciousness, memory disturbance, or twilight states, phenomena frequently observed in hysteria or epilepsy. Others are characterized by restless, nomadic tendencies, deserting repeatedly and with awareness, their actions suffused with latent hostility toward paternal authority. In these cases, Tausk interprets desertion as a displacement of aggression originally directed at the father or other authority figures—teachers, superiors—now projected onto the military as a symbolic paternal substitute.

He also includes those who desert out of fear of punishment after committing infractions, as well as those unable to endure the physical or psychological demands of military life. Another group comprises neurotic individuals afflicted by obsessive thoughts and anxiety-laden ideation, consistent with the metapsychology of neurosis outlined by Freud. Still others, he argues, desert as a form of psychic regression: fleeing not merely from the battlefield, but toward an earlier, more gratifying stage of life, seeking maternal protection through symbolic substitutes such as romantic partners. Tausk further notes the existence of "political deserters"—those whose refusal to fight is motivated by ideological conviction—and finally, those guided by moral, religious, or philosophical scruples who reject war on ethical grounds.

An illustrative example is provided through the case of a German soldier who deserted from Warsaw to Lublin after contracting gonorrhea. This young man feared retribution from his captain, who had issued severe threats regarding venereal infections. Through psychoanalytic inquiry, Tausk traced this anxiety to early traumatic experiences with an alcoholic and violent father who regularly abused his wife and children. The soldier's terror of punitive authority thus represented not rational apprehension, but the repetition of a deeply entrenched unconscious configuration, a return of the repressed in the form of pathological obedience and fear.

Regarding neurotic deserters, Tausk proposes that their inability to face the rigors of military life precipitates a regression to an infantile state characterized by dependence on maternal figures. Such individuals, he maintains, have failed to achieve full psychic separation from the maternal imago and remain fixated at a pre-oedipal stage of development. Their desertion, therefore, is less a conscious act of defiance than an expression of the ego's failure to sustain adult autonomy in the face of anxiety and external threat.

This psychoanalytic reading culminates in a powerful critique of prevailing legal conceptions of responsibility. According to military law, a crime is punishable only when committed freely and with full awareness of its consequences. This principle, Tausk contends, rests on the false assumption that human actions are wholly conscious and rationally motivated. Psychoanalysis, by contrast, reveals that unconscious motives—by definition inaccessible to conscious reflection—exert a determining influence on behavior. To equate such actions with deliberate, intentional conduct is, therefore, a profound misjudgment. For Tausk, the unconscious must be acknowledged as a legitimate causal force in human affairs, necessitating a fundamental rethinking of culpability and accountability.

In proposing this paradigm shift, Tausk not only anticipates the later development of forensic psychoanalysis but also prefigures an entire strand of twentieth-century thought concerned with the limits of legal rationality. His call for a "psychological reform of justice" situates him among the first to articulate a psychoanalytic critique of juridical systems that exclude the unconscious as a determinant of conduct. Ferenczi would later expand on these ideas, extending their relevance far beyond the military to encompass a broader spectrum of socially regulated behaviors.

Metapsychological Reflections on Repression and Other Defenses

Closely related to these considerations is Tausk's essay "Compensation as a means of discounting the motive of repression" (Tausk, 1913a/1983a), a subtle and theoretically sophisticated work in which he examines the mechanisms by which repressed ideas may lose their affective charge and thereby emerge into consciousness without provoking anxiety or resistance. Within the analytic process—particularly through the technique of free association—the chain of associations produced by the patient reveals the unconscious determinants underlying specific behaviors. A key aspect of this process, according to Tausk, is identifying a motive capable of explaining the displacement of affect from one representation to another.

Tausk argues that the displacement of affect entails a psychological correlate of devaluation. Through this mechanism, experiences that would ordinarily be felt as painful, humiliating, or shameful are stripped of emotional intensity, as their libidinal investment—cathexis—is transferred to a neutral representation. The original content thus loses its capacity to generate distress, having been rendered affectively inert.

Of particular relevance to Tausk are two clinical populations: individuals suffering from early-onset dementia—which he considered a precursor of schizophrenia—and those exhibiting paranoid traits. In the first group, unpleasant affects are displaced in such a way that the patient's associative productions appear emotionally flat or indifferent. The repressed emotion has been transferred to a symbolic substitute, allowing the ego to maintain untroubled contact with reality and shielding it from the full impact of conflict. In contrast, paranoid individuals deploy a distinct defensive strategy: rather than neutralizing their repressed contents intrapsychically, they project them outward, attributing to external agents the impulses and affects they cannot acknowledge in themselves. This mechanism, projection, generates a distorted perception of reality wherein others are experienced as harboring precisely the motives the subject repudiates.

Through this analysis, Tausk delineates the metapsychological boundaries separating neurotic from psychotic modes of functioning. In neurosis, repression and displacement act as internal regulators, preserving psychic balance by diverting anxiety-inducing content into tolerable forms. In psychosis, by contrast, the failure of repression results in a radical externalization of conflict: reality itself becomes the stage upon which the disowned elements of the psyche are re-enacted. The ego's relation to reality is thus transformed from a mediated to a persecutory one.

In articulating these distinctions, Tausk ventured into theoretical territory that remained largely peripheral to Freud's early metapsychology. Yet his reflections anticipated later developments in ego psychology, object relations theory, and the psychoanalytic study of psychosis. His writings on compensation, repression, and projection reveal a mind deeply engaged with the structural dynamics of the psyche and its defensive configurations—concerns that would resonate throughout twentieth-century psychoanalytic thought.

With these final reflections, this chapter comes to a close. What follows is a reflective Afterword and a detailed "Chronology of Viktor Tausk's life and work"—a brief yet incandescent trajectory that continues to illuminate the intersections of psychoanalysis, psychopathology, and the fragile architecture of the human mind.

Afterword

As traced throughout the pages of this book, the story of Viktor Tausk is compelling not only on a human level but also as a privileged vantage point from which to observe the institutional, affective, and theoretical tensions that shaped the early psychoanalytic movement. His life—and its tragic end—lay bare the vulnerabilities interwoven into the very fabric of psychoanalysis itself: the fragile balance between authority and innovation, between fidelity and individuation, between the rigor of theory and the unruly vitality of emotional life.

Tausk thus emerges not as a peripheral figure orbiting the Freudian sun, but as a vital interlocutor—one whose questions, conflicts, and insights continue to reverberate across time. His intellectual audacity, combined with an extraordinary emotional sensitivity, exposes the personal and collective costs of belonging to a movement that demanded unqualified allegiance, even as it struggled to define its own evolving identity.

In the drama that was his life, Tausk's path ultimately turned—irreversibly—toward *Thanatos*, at the expense of *Eros*. It was not the instinct for life that marked his final gesture, but rather a surrender to despair, which had by then assumed the weight and inevitability of illness. Suicide, for Tausk, appeared not as rebellion but as release—the only conceivable escape from psychic torment. He died as he had lived: a man of great intensity, divided by contradictions he could no longer reconcile.

Here, one recalls the aphorism of the pre-Socratic philosopher Heraclitus: *êthos anthrôpô daimôn*—"character is destiny." Heraclitus meant that it is through our inner disposition, our pattern of being, that our fate unfolds. And yet Tausk, who more than most understood—through both theory and clinical practice—the decisive role of the unconscious in human life, could not entirely avert a destiny that, in the end, was a reconfiguration of his own psychic truth. His fate was not a moral failure, but a tragic testament to the limits of self-knowledge when the unconscious asserts its sovereignty.

His struggle evokes a symbolic labyrinth—a modern Daedalian maze whose inescapable Minotaur was the embodied force of his inner conflict. Unlike Daedalus or his son Icarus, Tausk did not seek to soar toward

DOI: 10.4324/9781003716426-6

transcendence or fall in pursuit of the sun; his flight was of another order—a descent, not an ascent. Yet psychoanalysis teaches that there is no true escape from the psyche's demands: what is disavowed returns, and what remains unconscious must eventually be brought into awareness if it is to be transformed. "Where id was, there ego shall be"—but in Tausk's case, the ego could not hold. His tragedy thus becomes emblematic of the very terrain he sought to understand: the fragile architecture of psychic integration.

And still, suicide leaves a residue—a haunting echo that reverberates across generations. It inscribes a silent question in the hearts of those left behind: *Could it have been otherwise?* For those who loved him, who believed that another path might have been possible, the question lingers like an open wound. Might a single word, a gesture of tenderness, or a moment of presence have tipped the balance toward life? The most poignant example is that of Marius Tausk, Viktor's eldest son, who visited his father on the evening of July 2, 1919, the day before his death (Roazen, 1990, p. 123). Seventeen years old and studying medicine in Graz, Marius immediately sensed his father's fragility. He stayed for nearly two hours—offering, one imagines, comfort, or perhaps simply the quiet companionship of filial devotion. As he rose to leave, Viktor said gently: "Never mind about me" ["Kümmere Dich nicht um mich"] (M. Tausk, 1973, p. 332; Eissler, 1983, p. 111). Yet, according to Robert Jan Maarten Tausk, Viktor's grandson, Marius departed deeply disturbed. Upon returning to Graz, he learned that his father had taken his life the following morning (R. J. M. Tausk, personal communication, September 2, 2025).

It is impossible not to feel the poignancy of that moment, even at a century's distance. One imagines the stillness, the unsaid words, the unbearable foreknowledge in the son's heart. This encounter, suspended between intimacy and loss, marks perhaps the most human point of the entire tragedy. The wound it opened in Marius could hardly have healed; time may have dulled its edges, but such pain never wholly disappears. It lingers, folded into memory, shaping the emotional texture of those who remain.

In writing this book, my aim has not been to reopen those wounds, nor to adjudicate the moral or historical disputes surrounding Freud or his circle. Rather, it has been to offer a historically grounded and intellectually faithful reconstruction of Tausk's life and work—to recover, as far as possible, the complexity of the man and the epoch that formed him. Above all, this study is meant as a gesture of fidelity: fidelity to his contradictions, to his brilliance, to the fragile humanity that animated his thought and shadowed his existence. To read Tausk is to confront the inseparability of insight and suffering, of lucidity and loss.

"The rest," as Jung wrote to Freud in their final letter of January 6, 1913, "is silence" (Freud & Jung, 1974/1978, p. 612). Jung used the phrase to mark the dissolution of their intellectual bond. Yet one cannot help but wonder what might have transpired between Freud and Tausk had the latter not succumbed to despair. That question, too, belongs now to the silence.

And so, to those who have accompanied me to this final page, I offer no definitive conclusion. Instead, I invite you to dwell briefly in that silence—to let its resonance speak within you, softly and inwardly. Perhaps there, beyond interpretation, something of Tausk's presence still endures—subtle, unresolved, but alive.

Chronology of Viktor Tausk's Life and Work

1879 Viktor Tausk is born on March 12 in Zsilina (now Žilina, Slovakia), into a Jewish family.

1897 Begins law studies at the University of Vienna.

1900 Marries Martha Frisch on May 13 and relocates to what was then Yugoslavia.

1902 His first son, Marius, is born. Tausk completes his law degree and earns a doctorate in jurisprudence.

1903 His second son, Victor Hugo, is born.

1905 Tausk and Martha separate and return independently to Vienna. That same year, he writes "Husein Brko: Bosnische Zigeunergroteske" [Husein Brko: A Bosnian gypsy grotesque] and "Halbdunkel" [Twilight].

1906 Moves to Berlin, where he begins working as a journalist.

1907 Admitted to a sanatorium for 25 days to treat a tuberculosis outbreak and a depressive episode. During his Berlin stay, he meets Lea Rosen and writes an essay on Spinoza.

1908 In October, he returns to Vienna, finalizes his divorce from Martha on the 20th, and enrolls in the University of Vienna's medical school.

1909 In October, he attends his first scientific meeting of the Vienna Psychoanalytic Society. On November 24, presents his first paper to the group: "Theory of knowledge and psychoanalysis."

1910 In March, the Second International Psychoanalytic Congress takes place in Nuremberg, Germany. Ferenczi proposes the founding of what will become the International Psychoanalytical Association (IPA).

1911 Amid this rift between Freud and Alfred Adler—which ultimately leads to Adler's departure from the Vienna Psychoanalytic Society and the founding, on May 14, of the Association for Free Psychoanalysis (later renamed the Association for Individual Psychology)—Tausk stands firmly with Freud. Just days earlier, on May 10, he had presented to the Vienna Psychoanalytic Society an oral communication titled "A contribution to the psychology of masochism." Later that year, on October 18, he returns to the Vienna Psychoanalytic

DOI: 10.4324/9781003716426-7

Society to present another paper, "Problems dealt with in and as a result of psychoanalysis."

1912 Publishes his essay "On masturbation" and presents two papers before the Vienna Psychoanalytic Society: "Sexuality and ego" on March 27, and "Two contributions to the psychoanalysis of the inhibition of artistic production" on November 27. Begins a romantic relationship with Lou Andreas-Salomé. Meanwhile, Helene Deutsch starts working at the Wagner-Jauregg Clinic in Vienna. The so-called "Secret Committee" is formed to shield Freud and psychoanalysis from internal dissent—particularly from Jung, whose departure is now imminent. A new journal, *Internationale Zeitschrift für ärztliche Psychoanalyse*, is launched with Freud as general editor and Ferenczi, Rank, and Jones as executive editors, marginalizing Wilhelm Stekel and the *Zentralblatt*. Freud's relationship with Jung continues to deteriorate.

1913 On March 12, Tausk presents his paper "The father problem" to the Vienna Psychoanalytic Society. That same year, he publishes several important contributions, including "Compensation as a means of discounting the motive of repression," "Depiction of the dreamer's situation within the dream," and "A contribution to the psychology of child sexuality." In addition, he writes two discerning critical reviews: one of Jan Nelken's "Analytical observations on the fantasies of a schizophrenic" and another of Shaina Grebelskaya's "Psychological analysis of a paranoid."

1914 In June, receives his medical degree. A few weeks later, the outbreak of World War I radically transforms the European landscape. Despite the upheaval, Tausk remains intellectually productive. He publishes "Two homosexual dreams," "A dream of numbers," "Short contributions to the interpretation of dreams," and "Psychoanalysis of philosophy and psychoanalytic philosophy." On December 30, presents to the Vienna Psychoanalytic Society his paper "Contributions to a psychoanalytic exposition of melancholia."

1915 In August, enlists in the military. Earlier that year, on March 31, presents to the Vienna Psychoanalytic Society his paper "On the psychology of alcoholic occupational delirium," which is subsequently published under the same title.

1916 On March 25, his father dies. That same year, he publishes "Diagnostic considerations concerning the symptomatology of the so-called war psychosis," "On the psychology of the war deserter," "On a particular form of obsessive fantasies," and "Contributions to the psychopathology of everyday life." In December, he is transferred from Lublin to Belgrade, where he begins a relationship with Kosa Lazarević.

1917 Publishes "Some comments on Abraham's paper on 'ejaculatio praecox.'"

1918 World War I ends. On September 28–29, the Fifth International Psychoanalytic Congress is held in Budapest, where Tausk presents his paper "Psychoanalysis and the capacity for judgment." On November 4, he returns to Vienna and resumes psychiatric practice. In December, Freud refuses to analyze Tausk himself and instead appoints Helene Deutsch—then still Freud's own analysand—to take on the task.

1919 In January, Tausk begins analysis with Deutsch, which is interrupted three months later under Freud's directive. That spring, he becomes engaged to Hilde Loewi, with their wedding set for mid-July. On the morning of July 3—just ten days before the planned ceremony—Tausk dies by suicide, both hanging himself and shooting himself in the head. His seminal paper "On the origin of the 'influencing machine' in schizophrenia" is published posthumously. Freud writes a formal obituary in his honor.

1934 His posthumous work "Contribution to the psychopathology of everyday life" is published.

1973 His literary critique of Gerhart Hauptmann's *Und Pippa tanzt* [And Pippa dances] is published in *American Imago*.

References

Abraham, K. (1917/1994). Eyaculación precoz. In K. Abraham, *Psicoanálisis clínico* (D. R. Wagner, Trans.; pp. 213–227). Lumen-Hormé. (Original work published 1917)

Andreas-Salomé, L. (1951/1988). *Mirada retrospectiva: Compendio de algunos recuerdos de la vida* (A. Venegas, Trans.). Alianza Editorial. (Original work published 1951)

Andreas-Salomé, L. (1958/1984). *Aprendiendo con Freud: Diario de un año 1912/1913* (L. Lalucat & J. Vehil, Trans.; 3rd ed.). Laertes. (Original work published 1958)

Appignanesi, L., & Forrester, J. (1992). *Freud's women*. Weidenfeld & Nicholson.

Bachofen, J. J. (1861). *Das Mutterrecht: Eine Untersuchung über die Gynaikokratie der alten Welt nach ihrer religiösen und rechtlichen Natur* [Mother right: An inquiry into the matriarchal structures of the ancient world according to their religious and legal character]. Krais & Hoffmann.

Baer, A. (1901). *Der Selbstmord im kindlichen Lebensalter* [Suicide in childhood]. G. Thieme.

Balbuena, F. (2020). Sabina Spielrein: From being a psychiatric patient to becoming an analyst herself. *American Journal of Psychoanalysis*, 80(3), 281–308. doi:10.1057/s11231-020-09260-0.

Bentinck van Schoonheten, A. (2013/2016). *Karl Abraham: Life and work, a biography* (L. Waters, Trans.). Karnac. (Original work published 2013)

Binion, R. (1968). *Frau Lou: Nietzsche's wayward disciple*. Princeton University Press.

Birman, J. (1990). *Tausk: O aparelho de influenciar na psicose*. Escuta.

Bleichmar, H. (1997). *Avances en psicoterapia psicoanalítica*. Paidós.

Breuer, J., & Freud, S. (1893–1895/1980). Estudios sobre la histeria. In S. Freud, *Obras completas* (J. L. Etcheverry, Trans.; Vol. 2, pp. 1–317). Amorrortu. (Original work published 1893–1895)

Burston, D. (2006). In memoriam: Paul Roazen (1936–2005). *American Imago*, 63(1), 109–118. www.jstor.org/stable/26305299.

Carotenuto, A., & Trombetta, C. (1981). *Sabina Spielrein entre Freud et Jung*. Aubier.

Casals, J. (2003). *Afinidades vienesas: Sujeto, lenguaje, arte*. Anagrama.

Clark, R. W. (1985/1980). *Freud: El hombre y su causa*. Planeta. (Original work published 1980)

Clark-Lowes, F. (2010). *Freud's apostle: Wilhelm Stekel and the early history of psychoanalysis*. Authors Online.

Corliss, C. (2018). *A primer of the psychoanalytic theory of Herbert Silberer: What Silberer said*. Routledge.

Deutsch, H. (1919). Ein kasuistischer Beitrag zur Kenntnis des Mechanismus der Regression bei Schizophrenie [A case-based contribution to the understanding of the mechanism of regression in schizophrenia]. *Internationale Zeitschrift für Psychoanalyse*, 5, 41–45.

Deutsch, H., & Roazen, P. (1985). A case that throws light on the mechanism of regression in schizophrenia. *Psychoanalytic Review*, 72(1), 1–8.

Die Onanie: Vierzehn Beiträge zu einer Diskussion der Wiener psychoanalytischen Vereinigung [On masturbation: Fourteen contributions to a discussion of the Vienna Psychoanalytic Society]. (1912). J. F. Bergmann.

Donat, B. (2007). Viktor Tausk, Sigmund Freud i hrvatska moderna okupljena oko zagrebačko bečkoga časopisa Mladost [Viktor Tausk, Sigmund Freud and the Croatian modernist movement around the Zagreb-Vienna journal Mladost]. *Književna republika: Časopis za književnost* (3–4), 68–88.

Dorfer, B. (2007). *Die Lebensreise der Martha Tausk: Sozialdemokratie und Frauenrechte im Brennpunkt* [The life journey of Martha Tausk: Social democracy and women's rights in focus]. Studien Verlag.

Dybel, P. (2020). *Psychoanalysis – the promised land? The history of psychoanalysis in Poland 1900–1989. Part I: The Sturm und Drang period. Beginnings of psychoanalysis in the Polish lands during the partitions 1900–1918* (T. Bieroń, Trans.; R. Nycz, Ed.; Cross-Roads: Polish Studies in Culture, Literary Culture, and History, Vol. 20). Peter Lang.

Eissler, K. R. (1971). *Talent and genius: The fictitious case of Tausk contra Freud*. Quadrangle.

Eissler, K. R. (1974). On misstatements of would-be Freud biographers with special reference to the Tausk controversy. *International Review of Psycho-Analysis*, 1, 391–414.

Eissler, K. R. (1983). *Victor Tausk's suicide*. International Universities Press.

Etkind, A. (1993/1997). *Eros of the impossible: The history of psychoanalysis in Russia* (N. Rubins & M. Rubins, Trans.). Westview Press. (Original work published 1993)

Falzeder, E., Brabant, E., & Giampieri-Deutsch, P. (with the collaboration of). (1994). *The correspondence of Sigmund Freud and Sándor Ferenczi* (Vol. 1, 1908–1914; P. T. Hoffer, Trans.). Harvard University Press.

Falzeder, E., Brabant, E., & Giampieri-Deutsch, P. (with the collaboration of). (1996). *The correspondence of Sigmund Freud and Sándor Ferenczi* (Vol. 2, 1914–1919; P. T. Hoffer, Trans.). Harvard University Press.

Farridnejad, S. (2016, July 6). Friedrich Carl Andreas: A man for all seasons. In *Bibliographia Iranica: Events*. Retrieved September 22, 2025, from www.biblioiranica.info/friedrich-carl-andreas-a-man-for-all-seasons.

Federn, E. (1973). Correspondence arising from the publication of Reflections on ethos and authenticity in psychoanalysis. *The Human Context*, 5(3), 676.

Ferenczi, S. (1908/1981a). Sobre el alcance de la eyaculación precoz. In S. Ferenczi, *Obras completas* (F. J. Aguirre, Trans.; Vol. 1, 1908–1912. *Psicoanálisis I*, pp. 15–18). Espasa-Calpe. (Original work published 1908)

Ferenczi, S. (1912/1981b). Filosofía y psicoanálisis. In S. Ferenczi, *Obras completas* (F. J. Aguirre, Trans.; Vol. 1, 1908–1912. *Psicoanálisis I*, pp. 249–257). Espasa-Calpe. (Original work published 1912)

Fliess, R. (Ed.). (1948). The psychoanalytic reader: An anthology of essential papers with critical introductions. International Universities Press.

Freiherr von Winterstein, A. (1913). Psychoanalytische Anmerkungen zur Geschichte der Philosophie [Psychoanalytic notes on the history of philosophy]. *Imago*, 2, 175–237.

Freud Museum. (n.d.). Karl Weiss (Weiß), Alfred von Winterstein – Bios Weiss – Winterstein. Freud Museum Vienna. Retrieved October 12, 2025, from www.freud-museum.at/en/subsites-organized-escape.

Freud, S. (1900/1979a). La interpretación de los sueños (primera parte) (1900). In S. Freud, *Obras completas* (J. L. Etcheverry, Trans.; Vol. 4, pp. 1–343). Amorrortu. (Original work published 1900)

Freud, S. (1900/1979b). La interpretación de los sueños (segunda parte). Sobre el sueño (1900–1901). In S. Freud, *Obras completas* (J. L. Etcheverry, Trans.; Vol. 5, pp. 345–747). Amorrortu. (Original work published 1900)

Freud, S. (1901/1980a). Psicopatología de la vida cotidiana. In S. Freud, *Obras completas* (J. L. Etcheverry, Trans.; Vol. 6, pp. 1–306). Amorrortu. (Original work published 1901)

Freud, S. (1905a/1978a). Tres ensayos de teoría sexual. In S. Freud, *Obras completas* (J. L. Etcheverry, Trans.; Vol. 7, pp. 109–224). Amorrortu. (Original work published 1905a)

Freud, S. (1905b/1978b). Fragmento de análisis de un caso de histeria. In S. Freud, *Obras completas* (J. L. Etcheverry, Trans.; Vol. 7, pp. 1–108). Amorrortu. (Original work published 1905b)

Freud, S. (1910/1979c). Las perspectivas futuras de la terapia psicoanalítica. In S. Freud, *Obras completas* (J. L. Etcheverry, Trans.; Vol. 11, pp. 129–142). Amorrortu. (Original work published 1910)

Freud, S. (1911/1980b). Puntualizaciones psicoanalíticas sobre un caso de paranoia descrito autobiográficamente. In S. Freud, *Obras completas* (J. L. Etcheverry, Trans.; Vol. 12, pp. 1–76). Amorrortu. (Original work published 1911)

Freud, S. (1912a/1980c). Sobre la dinámica de la transferencia. In S. Freud, *Obras completas* (J. L. Etcheverry, Trans.; Vol. 12, pp. 93–105). Amorrortu. (Original work published 1912a)

Freud, S. (1912b/1980d). Consejos al médico sobre el tratamiento psicoanalítico. In S. Freud, *Obras completas* (J. L. Etcheverry, Trans.; Vol. 12, pp. 107–119). Amorrortu. (Original work published 1912b)

Freud, S. (1913/1980e). Tótem y tabú. In S. Freud, *Obras completas* (J. L. Etcheverry, Trans.; Vol. 13, pp. 1–164). Amorrortu. (Original work published 1913)

Freud, S. (1914a/1979d). Contribución a la historia del movimiento psicoanalítico. In S. Freud, *Obras completas* (J. L. Etcheverry, Trans.; Vol. 14, pp. 1–64). Amorrortu. (Original work published 1914a)

Freud, S. (1914b/1979e). Introducción del narcisismo. In S. Freud, *Obras completas* (J. L. Etcheverry, Trans.; Vol. 14, pp. 65–98). Amorrortu. (Original work published 1914b)

Freud, S. (1914c/1980f). Recordar, repetir y reelaborar. In S. Freud, *Obras completas* (J. L. Etcheverry, Trans.; Vol. 12, pp. 145–157). Amorrortu. (Original work published 1914c)

Freud, S. (1917/1979f). Duelo y melancolía. In S. Freud, *Obras completas* (J. L. Etcheverry, Trans.; Vol. 14, pp. 235–258). Amorrortu. (Original work published 1917)

Freud, S. (1919/1979g). Victor Tausk. In S. Freud, *Obras completas* (J. L. Etcheverry, Trans.; Vol. 17, pp. 266–268). Amorrortu. (Original work published 1919)

Freud, S. (1920/1979h). Más allá del principio de placer. In S. Freud, *Obras completas* (J. L. Etcheverry, Trans.; Vol. 18, pp. 1–62). Amorrortu. (Original work published 1920)

Freud, S. (1927/1979i). Fetichismo. In S. Freud, *Obras completas* (J. L. Etcheverry, Trans.; Vol. 21, pp. 141–152). Amorrortu. (Original work published 1927)

Freud, S. (1936/1979j). Carta a Romain Rolland (Una perturbación del recuerdo en la Acrópolis). In S. Freud, *Obras completas* (J. L. Etcheverry, Trans.; Vol. 22, pp. 209–221). Amorrortu. (Original work published 1936)

Freud, S. (1937/1980g). Análisis terminable e interminable. In S. Freud, *Obras completas* (J. L. Etcheverry, Trans.; Vol. 23, pp. 211–254). Amorrortu. (Original work published 1937)

Freud, S., & Abraham, K. (1965/1979). *Correspondencia.* Gedisa. (Original work published 1965)

Freud, S., & Andreas-Salomé, L. (1966/1968). *Correspondencia.* Siglo XXI. (Original work published 1966)

Freud, S., & Jung, C. G. (1974/1978). *Correspondencia* (W. McGuire & W. Sauerländer, Eds.; A. Guéra Miralles, Trans.). Taurus. (Original work published 1974)

Freud, S., & Pfister, O. (1963/1966). *Correspondencia: 1909–1933.* Fondo de Cultura Económica. (Original work published 1963)

Gavin, J. (2017, February 9). Kurt R. Eissler and the Sigmund Freud Archives. Timeless: Stories from the Library. Library of Congress. Retrieved August 4, 2025, from https://blogs.loc.gov/loc/2017/02/kurt-r-eissler-and-the-sigmund-freud-archives/.

Gay, P. (1988). *Freud: A life for our time.* W. W. Norton & Company.

Gebsattel, V. E. von. (1912). Der Einzelne und der Zuschauer: Untersuchung zur Psychologie und Pathologie des Triebes nach Beachtung [The individual and the spectator: An inquiry into the psychology and pathology of the drive for attention] (pp. 36–78). *Zeitschrift für Pathopsychologie.* Verlag von Wilhelm Engelmann.

Gelfand, T., & Kerr, J. (2013). *Freud and the history of psychoanalysis.* Routledge.

Goethe, J. W. von. (1774). *Die Leiden des jungen Werthers* [The sorrows of young Werther]. Weygand'sche Buchhandlung.

González, A. (1997). *El pensamiento filosófico de Lou Andreas-Salomé.* Cátedra.

Grebelskaja, S. (1912). Psychologische Analyse eines Paranoiden [Psychological analysis of a paranoid]. *Jahrbuch für psychoanalytische und psychopathologische Forschungen*, 4, 116–140.

Grenville, A. (2012, July). The case of Gerhart Hauptmann. *AJR Journal (Association of Jewish Refugees)*, 12(7), 1–2.

Grimm, J., & Grimm, W. (1812). *Kinder- und Hausmärchen* [Children's and household tales] (Bd. 1). Realschulbuchhandlung.

Grotjahn, M. (1991). Introduction. In E. Weiss, *Sigmund Freud as a consultant: Recollections of a pioneer in psychoanalysis* (pp. xiii–xix). Transaction Publishers.

Grotjahn, M., & Illing, H. A. (1966/1968). Victor Tausk: La máquina de influencia. In M. Grotjahn *et al.*, *Historia del psicoanálisis*, IV (R. Baretto, Trans.; pp. 11–17). Paidós. (Original work published 1966)

Grosskurth, P. (1986). *Melanie Klein: Her world and her work.* Hodder & Stoughton.

Grubrich-Simitis, I. (1991). Histoire de l'édition des œuvres de Freud en langue allemande. *Revue Internationale d'Histoire de la Psychanalyse*, 4, 13–70.

Guillerault, G. (1974). L'étrange histoire du disciple aimé et détesté de Freud. *Psychologie*, 58, 15–23.

Gutheil, E. A. (Ed.). (1950). *The autobiography of Wilhelm Stekel: The life story of a pioneer psychoanalyst.* Liveright.

Hamilton, J. W. (1991). A reconsideration of the Freud–Tausk–Deutsch relationship. *Psychoanalytic Review*, 78(2), 267–278.

Heilbronner, K. (1903). Ueber Fugues und fugue-ähnliche Zustände [On fugues and fugue-related states]. *Jahrbücher für Psychiatrie und Neurologie*, 23, 107–206.

Hitschmann, E. (1913). Schopenhauer: Versuch einer Psychoanalyse des Philosophen [An attempt at a psychoanalysis of the philosopher]. *Imago*, 2, 101–174.

Hugo, V. (1829). *Le dernier jour d'un condamné* [The last day of a condemned man]. Charles Gosselin.

Jekels, L. (n.d.). *Early psychoanalytic reminiscences* [Unpublished manuscript]. Siegfried Bernfeld Papers (Container 17), Library of Congress, Washington, DC.

JewAge.org. (2008–2025). Pavel Nahumovitch Sheftel [Biographical profile]. Retrieved August 18, 2025, from www.jewage.org/wiki/en/Profile:P0678266441.

Jones, E. (1911). Review of Die Sprache des Traumes. Eine Darstellung der Symbolik und Deutung des Traumes in ihren Beziehungen zur kranken und gesunden Seele für Ärzte und Psychologen [Review of the book Die Sprache des Traumes. Eine Darstellung der Symbolik und Deutung des Traumes in ihren Beziehungen zur kranken und gesunden Seele für Ärzte und Psychologen, by W. Stekel]. *The Journal of Abnormal Psychology*, 6(4), 327–328. doi:10.1037/h0068764.

Jones, E. (1953). *The life and work of Sigmund Freud (Vol. 1, The formative years and the great discoveries, 1856–1900)*. Basic Books.

Jones, E. (1955). *The life and work of Sigmund Freud (Vol. 2, Years of maturity, 1901–1919)*. Basic Books.

Jones, E. (1957). *The life and work of Sigmund Freud (Vol. 3, The last phase, 1919–1939)*. Basic Books.

Jung, C. G. (1912). *Wandlungen und Symbole der Libido: Beiträge zur Entwicklungsgeschichte des Denkens* [Transformations and symbols of the libido: Contributions to the history of the development of thought]. Sonderabdruck aus dem Jahrbuch für psychoanalytische und psychopathologische Forschungen (Bd. 3–4).

Jung, C. G. (1913). Eine Bemerkung zur Tauskschen Kritik der Nelkenschen Arbeit [A remark on Tausk's critique of Nelken's work]. *Internationale Zeitschrift für Psychoanalyse*, 1, 285–288.

Kanzer, M. (1971). An autobiographical legacy of Victor Tausk. *International Journal of Psychoanalysis*, 52, 423–430.

Kanzer, M. (1972). Victor Tausk: The creativity and suicide of a psychoanalyst. *Psychoanalytic Quarterly*, 41(4), 556–584.

Kanzer, M. (1973a). Comment on the letter of Professor Marius Tausk. *American Imago*, 30(4), 336–339.

Kanzer, M. (1973b). Victor Tausk: Analyst and dramatic critic. *American Imago*, 30(4), 371–379.

Katyn Foundation. (2025). Jan Nelken [Families of Jewish Origin]. *Katyn Jews*. Retrieved September 30, 2025, from https://katynjews.com/tombstones/jan-nelken/.

Keller, G. (1855). *Der grüne Heinrich* [Green Henry] (1st ed.). Vieweg Verlag.

Keller, G. (1880). *Der grüne Heinrich* [Green Henry] (Revised ed.). Verlag Göschen.

Kern, S. (1973). Freud and the discovery of child sexuality. *History of Childhood Quarterly*, 1(1), 117–141.

Kerr, J. (1993). *A most dangerous method: The story of Jung, Freud, and Sabina Spielrein*. Alfred A. Knopf.

Lally, K. (2024). *Toward an emergent psychoanalysis: Thinking difference through the work of Victor Tausk* (Doctoral dissertation, University of California, Santa Cruz). eScholarship. https://escholarship.org/uc/item/2jd4m0zq.

Launer, J. (2014). *Sex versus survival: The life and ideas of Sabina Spielrein*. Duckworth Overlook.

Lewin, B. D. (1950). Paul Federn 1872–1950. *Psychoanalytic Quarterly*, 19(3), 295–297. doi:10.1080/21674086.1950.11925804.

Livingstone, A. (1984/1990). *Lou Andreas-Salomé: Sa vie et ses écrits* (P.-E. Dauzat, Trans.). Presses Universitaires de France. (Original work published 1984)

Löwenfeld, L. (1911). *Über die sexuelle Konstitution und andere Sexual-Probleme* [On the sexual constitution and other sex problems]. Bergmann.

Makari, G. (2008). *Revolution in mind: The creation of psychoanalysis*. Gerald Duckworth & Co. Ltd.

Malcolm, J. (1981). *Psychoanalysis: The impossible profession*. Alfred A. Knopf.

Malcolm, J. (1984). *In the Freud archives*. Alfred A. Knopf.

Marcinowski, J. (1909). Zur Frage der infantilen Sexualität [On the question of infantile sexuality]. *Berliner Klinische Wochenschrift*, 20, 927–928.

Marías, J. (1941/1970). *Historia de la filosofía*. Editorial Revista de Occidente. (Original work published 1941)

Masotta, O. (1983). Introducción. In V. Tausk (1983a), *Trabajos psicoanalíticos* (pp. 9–12). Gedisa.

Moellenhoff, F. (1966/1968). Hanns Sachs: El inconsciente creador. In H. Zulliger et al., *Historia del psicoanálisis*, III (N. Rosenblatt, Trans.; pp. 37–66). Paidós. (Original work published 1966)

Nelken, J. (1912). Analytische Beobachtungen über Phantasien eines Schizophrenen [Analytical observations on the fantasies of a schizophrenic]. *Jahrbuch für psychoanalytische und psychopathologische Forschungen*, 4(1), 504–562.

Neumarkt, P. (1973). Hauptmann's and Pippa dances and Victor Tausk's commentary. *American Imago*, 30(4), 360–370.

Neumarkt, P. (1977). The Freud-Tausk controversy: A symphony of disharmony. *International Review of Psychoanalysis*, 4, 363–373.

Neyant-Sutterman, T. (1978). Entretien avec Marius Tausk à Nimègue (mi-décembre 1978). *Revue Française de Psychanalyse*, 42, 747–751.

Nunberg, H., & Federn, E. (Eds.). (1962). *Minutes of the Vienna Psychoanalytic Society (Vol. 1, 1906–1908)* (M. Nunberg, Trans.). International Universities Press.

Nunberg, H., & Federn, E. (Eds.). (1967). *Minutes of the Vienna Psychoanalytic Society (Vol. 2, 1908–1910)* (M. Nunberg, Trans.). International Universities Press.

Nunberg, H., & Federn, E. (Eds.). (1974). *Minutes of the Vienna Psychoanalytic Society (Vol. 3, 1910–1911)* (M. Nunberg, Trans.). International Universities Press.

Nunberg, H., & Federn, E. (Eds.). (1975). *Minutes of the Vienna Psychoanalytic Society (Vol. 4, 1912–1918)* (M. Nunberg, Trans.). International Universities Press.

Orange, D. M., Atwood, G. E., & Stolorow, R. D. (1997). *Working intersubjectively: Contextualism in psychoanalytic practice*. The Analytic Press.

Österreichische Akademie der Wissenschaften [ÖAW]. (2022). Reinhold, Josef (1885–1947). In *Österreichisches Biographisches Lexikon (ÖBL)*. Austrian Centre for Digital Humanities and Cultural Heritage. Retrieved October 6, 2025 from www.biographien.ac.at/oebl/oebl_R/Reinhold_Josef_1885_1947.xml.

Peters, H. F. (1962/1995). *Lou Andreas-Salomé: Mi hermana, mi esposa* (A. M. de la Fuente, Trans.). Paidós. (Original work published 1962)

Petlevski, S. (2011). Zaboravljeno lice Moderne: Viktor Tausk kao dramatičar [The forgotten face of Modernism: Viktor Tausk as a playwright]. In B. Hećimović (Ed.),

Naši i strani povjesničari hrvatske drame i kazališta, teatrolozi i kritičari: Prvi dio: U spomen Nikoli Batušiću / Krležini dani u Osijeku 2010 [Our and foreign historians of Croatian drama and theatre, theatre scholars and critics: First part: In memory of Nikola Batušić / Krleža Days in Osijek 2010] (pp. 67–78). Hrvatska akademija znanosti i umjetnosti (HAZU).

Pfeiffer, E. (1958/1984). Prólogo. In L. Andreas-Salomé, *Aprendiendo con Freud: Diario de un año 1912/1913* (L. Lalucat & J. Vehil, Trans., 3rd ed., pp. 7–16). Laertes. (Original work published 1958)

Postone, M. (1980). Anti-semitism and national socialism: Notes on the German reaction to "Holocaust." *New German Critique* (19), 97–115.

Psychoanalytikerinnen in der Schweiz. (2025, July 14). Scheina (Jenny) Grebelskaja. *Psychoanalytikerinnen in der Schweiz. Biografisches Lexikon*. Retrieved October 7, 2025 from www.psychoanalytikerinnen.de/schweiz_biografien.html#Grebelskaja.

Putnam, J. (1912). The role of philosophical views and training in the further development of the psychoanalytic movement. *Imago*, 1, 101–118.

Randall, J. H., Jr. (1919). The problem in Wilbrandt's Meister von Palmyra . *Modern Philology*, 17(2), 57–76. www.jstor.org/stable/433199.

Rank, O., & Sachs, H. (1913). *Die Bedeutung der Psychoanalyse für die Geisteswissenschaften* [The significance of psychoanalysis for the humanities]. Bergmann.

Reich, W. (1921–1922). Der Koitus und die Geschlechter [Coition and the sexes]. *Zeitschrift für Sexualwissenschaft*, 8, 343–352.

Reich, W. (1926/1984). Los padres como educadores: La compulsión a educar y sus causas. In W. Reich & V. Schmidt, *Psicoanálisis y educación* (pp. 145–160). Orbis. (Original work published 1926)

Roazen, P. (1969). *Brother animal: The story of Freud and Tausk*. Alfred A. Knopf.

Roazen, P. (1969/1973). *Hermano animal: La historia de Freud y Tausk* (J. Rábago, Trans.). Alianza Editorial. (Original work published 1969)

Roazen, P. (1971/1978a). *Freud y sus discípulos* (C. Manzano, Trans.). Alianza Editorial. (Original work published in 1971)

Roazen, P. (1972). Reflections on ethos and authenticity in psychoanalysis. *The Human Context*, 4(3), 577–587.

Roazen, P. (1977). Orthodoxy on Freud: The case of Tausk. *Contemporary Psychoanalysis*, 13(1), 102–115.

Roazen, P. (1978b). Reading, writing, and memory: Dr. K. R. Eissler's thinking. *Contemporary Psychoanalysis*, 14(2), 345–353.

Roazen, P. (1980). *Victor Tausk, disciple of Sigmund Freud (Historical Perspectives on Depression, No. 6)*. The Professional Services Department of Roche Laboratories.

Roazen, P. (1982). On errors regarding Freud. *International Journal of Psychoanalysis*, 63, 260–261.

Roazen, P. (1990). *Brother animal: The story of Freud and Tausk* (2nd ed., with a new introduction). Transaction Publishers.

Roazen, P. (Ed.). (1991). *Sexuality, war, and schizophrenia: Collected psychoanalytic papers* (E. Mosbacher & others, Trans.). Transaction Publishers. (Original works by Victor Tausk)

Roazen, P. (1992). *Helen Deutsch: A psychoanalyst's life*. Transaction Publishers.

Roazen, P. (2005). *Edoardo Weiss: The house that Freud built*. Transaction Publishers.

Roazen, P. (Ed.). (2017a). *Sexuality, war, and schizophrenia: Collected psychoanalytic papers* (E. Mosbacher & others, Trans.). Routledge. (Original works by Victor Tausk)

Roazen, P. (2017b). Introduction. In P. Roazen (Ed.), *Sexuality, war, and schizophrenia: Collected psychoanalytic papers* (E. Mosbacher & others, Trans.; pp. 1–31). Routledge. (Original works by Victor Tausk)

Roazen, P., & Swerdloff, B. (1977). *Heresy: Sándor Radó and the psychoanalytic movement*. Jason Aronson Publishers.

Rodrigué, E. (1996). *Sigmund Freud. El siglo del psicoanálisis* (2 vols.). Editorial Sudamericana.

Roudinesco, E., & Plon, M. (1997). *Dictionnaire de la psychanalyse*. Fayard.

Rousseau, J.-J. (1761). *Julie ou la nouvelle Héloïse* [Julie, or the new Heloise]. Marc-Michel Rey.

Rudnytsky, P. L. (1987). *Freud and Oedipus*. Columbia University Press.

Sachs, H. (1933). The delay of the machine age. *Psychoanalytic Quarterly*, 2, 404–424.

Sade, D. A. F., Marquis de. (1971/1995). *Justine, ou les malheurs de la vertu* [Justine, or The misfortunes of virtue]. Gallimard. (Original work published in 1791)

Sade, D. A. F., Marquis de. (1979/1998). *La nouvelle Justine ou les malheurs de la vertu* [The new Justine]. Gallimard. (Original work published in 1797)

Sadger, J. (1913a). Über das Unbewußte und die Träume bei Hebbel [On the unconscious and the dreams of Hebbel]. *Imago*, 2, 336–356.

Sadger, J. (1913b). Freudsche Mechanismen bei Hebbel [Freudian mechanisms in Hebbel]. *Internationale Zeitschrift für Psychoanalyse*, 1, 165–168.

Sadger, J. (1920). *Friedrich Hebbel: Ein psychoanalytischer Versuch* [Friedrich Hebbel: A psychoanalytic study]. Franz Deuticke.

Sánchez-Barranco, A. (1996). *El psicoanálisis freudiano*. Repiso Libros.

Sánchez-Barranco, A., & Balbuena, F. (1998). *Vida y obra de Viktor Tausk: Un psicoanalista maldito* [The life and work of Viktor Tausk: A cursed psychoanalyst]. Repiso Libros.

Sauerteig, L. D. H. (2012). Loss of innocence: Albert Moll, Sigmund Freud and the invention of childhood sexuality around 1900. *Medical History*, 56(2), 156–183. doi:10.1017/mdh.2011.31.

Schur, M. (1972). *Freud: Living and dying*. International Universities Press.

Sperber, H. (1912). Über den Einfluß sexueller Momente auf Entstehung und Entwicklung der Sprache [On the influence of sexual factors on the origin and development of language]. *Imago*, 1, 405–453.

Sperber, M. A. (1972). Freud, Tausk, and the Nobel Prize complex. *Psychoanalytic Review*, 59(2), 283–293.

Spielrein, S. (1911). Über den psychologischen Inhalt eines Falles von Schizophrenie (dementia praecox) [On the psychological content of a case of schizophrenia (dementia praecox)]. *Jahrbuch für psychoanalytische und psychopathologische Forschungen*, 3(1), 329–400.

Spielrein, S. (1912). Die Destruktion als Ursache des Werdens [Destruction as the cause of coming into being]. *Jahrbuch für Psychanalytische und Psychopathologische Forschungen*, 4(1), 465–503.

Stanton, M. (1991). *Sándor Ferenczi: Reconsidering active intervention*. Free Association Books.

Stekel, W. (1911). *Die Sprache des Traumes. Eine Darstellung der Symbolik und Deutung des Traumes in ihren Beziehungen zur kranken und gesunden Seele für Ärzte und Psychologen* [The language of dreams. A presentation for physicians and psychologists of the interpretation and symbolism of the dream in its relation to both the sick and healthy mind]. Bergmann.

Stekel, W. (1922). *Sex and dreams: The language of dreams.* Badger.

Stekel, W. (1943). *The interpretation of dreams.* Liveright.

Sterba, R. F. (1985). *Reminiscences of a Viennese psychoanalyst.* Wayne State University Press.

Swoboda, H. (1904). *Die Perioden des menschlichen Organismus in ihrer psychologischen und biologischen Bedeutung* [The periods of the human organism in their psychological and biological significance]. Franz Deuticke.

Tausk, H. (1889). *Židovsko Pitanje* [The Jewish question]. Tiskarski Zavod Narodnih Novina.

Tausk, M. (1973). Victor Tausk as seen by his son. *American Imago*, 30(4), 323–335.

Tausk, M. (1983). Comment. In K. Eissler, *Victor Tausk's suicide* (pp. 299–322). International Universities Press.

Tausk, V. [Slovačić, V.]. (1897). Sivo oko [Gray eye]. *Nada: Pouci, zabavi i umjetnosti*, 3(13), 245.

Tausk, V. [Slovačić, V.]. (1898a). Zimsko cvijeće [Winter flowers]. *Nada: Pouci, zabavi i umjetnosti*, 4(7), 105.

Tausk, V. [Slovačić, V.]. (1898b). *A. Tresić-Pavičić kao liričar: Studija* [Dr. Ante Tresić Pavičić as a lyricist: A study]. F. Bogović.

Tausk, V. (1912/1983a). El onanismo. In V. Tausk, *Trabajos psicoanalíticos* (pp. 17–42). Gedisa. (Original work published 1912)

Tausk, V. (1913a). Analytische Beobachtungen über Phantasien eines Schizophrenen [Analytical observations on the fantasies of a schizophrenic]. *Internationale Zeitschrift für Psychoanalyse*, 1, 84–87.

Tausk, V. (1913b). Sch. Grebelskaja: Psychologische Analyse eines Paranoiden [Sch. Grebelskaja: Psychological analysis of a paranoid]. *Internationale Zeitschrift für Psychoanalyse*, 1, 88.

Tausk, V. (1913c/1983a). Desvalorización del motivo de la represión por recompensa. In V. Tausk, *Trabajos psicoanalíticos* (pp. 71–82). Gedisa. (Original work published 1913c)

Tausk, V. (1913d/1983a). Representación en el sueño de la postura del durmiente. In V. Tausk, *Trabajos psicoanalíticos* (p. 83). Gedisa. (Original work published 1913d)

Tausk, V. (1913e/1983a). Contribución a la psicología de la sexualidad infantil. In V. Tausk, *Trabajos psicoanalíticos* (pp. 85–103). Gedisa. (Original work published 1913e)

Tausk, V. (1914a). Psychoanalyse der Philosophie und psychoanalytische Philosophie [Psychoanalysis of philosophy and psychoanalytic philosophy]. *Jahrbuch für psychoanalytische und psychopathologische Forschungen*, 6, 405–412.

Tausk, V. (1914b/1983a). Dos sueños homosexuales. In V. Tausk, *Trabajos psicoanalíticos* (pp. 105–110). Gedisa. (Original work published 1914b)

Tausk, V. (1914c/1983a). Un sueño de cifras. In V. Tausk, *Trabajos psicoanalíticos* (pp. 111–113). Gedisa. (Original work published 1914c)

Tausk, V. (1914d/1983a). Breves contribuciones a la interpretación de los sueños. In V. Tausk, *Trabajos psicoanalíticos* (pp. 115–119). Gedisa. (Original work published 1914d)

Tausk, V. (1915/1983a). A propósito de la psicología del delirio de acción de los alcohólicos. In V. Tausk, *Trabajos psicoanalíticos* (pp. 43–70). Gedisa. (Original work published 1915)

Tausk, V. (1916a/1983a). Una forma particular de fantasías obsesivas. In V. Tausk, *Trabajos psicoanalíticos* (pp. 121–123). Gedisa. (Original work published 1916a)

Tausk, V. (1916b/1983a). Contribuciones a la psicopatología de la vida cotidiana. In V. Tausk, *Trabajos psicoanalíticos* (pp. 125–129). Gedisa. (Original work published 1916b)

Tausk, V. (1916c/1983a). Contribución a la psicología del desertor. In V. Tausk, *Trabajos psicoanalíticos* (pp. 131–159). Gedisa. (Original work published 1916c)

Tausk, V. (1917/1983a). Observaciones sobre el ensayo de Abraham "La eyaculación precoz." In V. Tausk, *Trabajos psicoanalíticos* (pp. 161–180). Gedisa. (Original work published 1917)

Tausk, V. (1919/1983a). Acerca de la génesis del aparato de influir en el curso de la esquizofrenia. In V. Tausk, *Trabajos psicoanalíticos* (pp. 181–221). Gedisa. (Original work published 1919)

Tausk, V. (1934a). Psychopathologie des Alltagslebens: Ibsen, der Apotheker [Psychopathology of everyday life: Ibsen the druggist]. *Almanach der Psychoanalyse*, 9, 161–166.

Tausk, V. (1934b). Ibsen the druggist (D. Feigenbaum, Trans.). *Psychoanalytic Quarterly*, 3(1), 137–141.

Tausk, V. (1934/1983a). Contribución a la psicología de la vida cotidiana. In V. Tausk, *Trabajos psicoanalíticos* (pp. 223–227). Gedisa. (Original work published 1934)

Tausk, V. (1973). Paraphrase as commentary and critique on Gerhart Hauptmann's and Pippa dances. *American Imago*, 30, 340–359.

Tausk, V. (1975). *Œuvres psychanalytiques* [Psychoanalytic works]. Payot.

Tausk, V. (1977). *Trabajos psicoanalíticos* [Psychoanalytic works]. Granica Editor.

Tausk, V. (1979). *Scritti psicoanalitici* [Psychoanalytic writings]. Astrolabio Ubaldini.

Tausk, V. (1983a). *Trabajos psicoanalíticos* [Psychoanalytic works]. Gedisa.

Tausk, V. (1983b). *Gesammelte psychoanalytische und literarische Schriften* [Collected psychoanalytic and literary writings]. Medusa.

Tréhel, G. (2006). Victor Tausk (1879–1919) et la médecine militaire. *L'Information Psychiatrique*, 82(3), 239–247.

Tréhel, G. (2011). Victor Tausk (1879–1919): Une théorisation des psychoses de guerre. *Perspectives Psy*, 50(2), 162–175.

Triarhou, L. C. (2018). Lothar von Frankl-Hochwart (1862–1914). *Journal of Neurology*, 265(12), 3036–3037. doi:10.1007/s00415-018-8757-3.

Urbach, K. (1921–1922). Über die zeitliche Gefühlsdifferenz während der Kohabitation [On the temporal difference of feelings during coitus]. *Zeitschrift für Sexualwissenschaft*, 8, 124–138.

Venier Alexander, I. (2015). *The life and times of Franz Alexander: From Budapest to California*. Karnac.

Venier Alexander, I. (2017). *Growing up Alexander: My life with a psychoanalytic pioneer*. Karnac.

Venier Alexander, I. (2025). *The lost legacy of Franz Alexander: A psychoanalytic pioneer revisited*. Karnac.

Weiss, E. (1932). Regression and projection in the superego. *International Journal of Psychoanalysis*, 13, 449–458.

Weiss, E. (1964). *Agoraphobia in the light of ego psychology*. Grune & Stratton.

Weiss, E. (1991). *Sigmund Freud as a consultant: Recollections of a pioneer in psychoanalysis.* Transaction Publishers.
Wilbrandt, A. (1896). *Der Meister von Palmyra: Dramatische Dichtung in fünf Aufzügen* [The master of Palmyra: A five-act dramatic poem] (5th ed.). J. G. Cotta.
Yorke, C. (1999, March 23). Kurt Eissler: Obituary. *The Guardian*. Retrieved September 2, 2025, from www.theguardian.com/news/1999/mar/23/guardianobituaries2.
Zola, É. (1899). *Fécondité* [Fecundity]. Bibliothèque Charpentier.

Index

For Product Safety Concerns and Information please contact our EU representative GPSR@taylorandfrancis.com
Taylor & Francis Verlag GmbH, Kaufingerstraße 24, 80331 München, Germany

www.ingramcontent.com/pod-product-compliance
Ingram Content Group UK Ltd.
Pitfield, Milton Keynes, MK11 3LW, UK
UKHW020004200926
475702UK00015B/2466

* 9 7 8 1 0 4 1 2 0 4 1 2 1 *